昆明学院学术著作丛书

香气对情绪及自主神经系统的影响——基于HRV的评估分析

Effects of Aroma on Emotions and Autonomic Nervous System: Based on Heart Rate Variability(HRV) Analysis and Assess

黄　琳

[西班牙] 路易斯·卡普迪维拉·奥古斯特 / 著

Lluís Capdevila Ortís

云南大学出版社

YUNNAN UNIVERSITY PRESS

图书在版编目（CIP）数据

香气对情绪及自主神经系统的影响：基于HRV的评估分析 = Effects of Aroma on Emotions and Autonomic Nervous System: Based on Heart Rate Variability (HRV) Analysis and Assess：英文、西班牙文 / 黄琳，(西) 路易斯 · 卡普迪维拉 · 奥古斯特著. -- 昆明：云南大学出版社，2019
（昆明学院学术著作丛书）
ISBN 978-7-5482-3711-2

Ⅰ. ①香… Ⅱ. ①黄… ②路… Ⅲ. ①香精油－疗法－研究－英文、西班牙文 Ⅳ. ①R459.9

中国版本图书馆CIP数据核字（2019）第123455号

策划编辑： 徐　曼
责任编辑： 陈桂华
封面设计： 周　旸

昆明学院学术著作丛书

香气对情绪及自主神经系统的影响——基于HRV的评估分析

Effects of Aroma on Emotions and Autonomic Nervous System: Based on Heart Rate Variability(HRV) Analysis and Assess

黄　琳
［西班牙］路易斯 · 卡普迪维拉 · 奥古斯特 / 著
Lluís Capdevila Ortís

出版发行： 云南大学出版社
印　　装： 昆明理煜印务有限公司
开　　本： 787mm × 1092mm　1/16
印　　张： 9（含彩插0.25印张）
字　　数： 171千
版　　次： 2019年12月第1版
印　　次： 2019年12月第1次印刷
书　　号： ISBN 978-7-5482-3711-2
定　　价： 42.00元

社　　址： 昆明市一二一大街182号（云南大学东陆校区英华园内）
邮　　编： 650091
电　　话：（0871）65031071　65033244
E-mail： market@ynup.com

若发现本书有印装质量问题，请与印厂联系调换，联系电话：0871- 64167045。

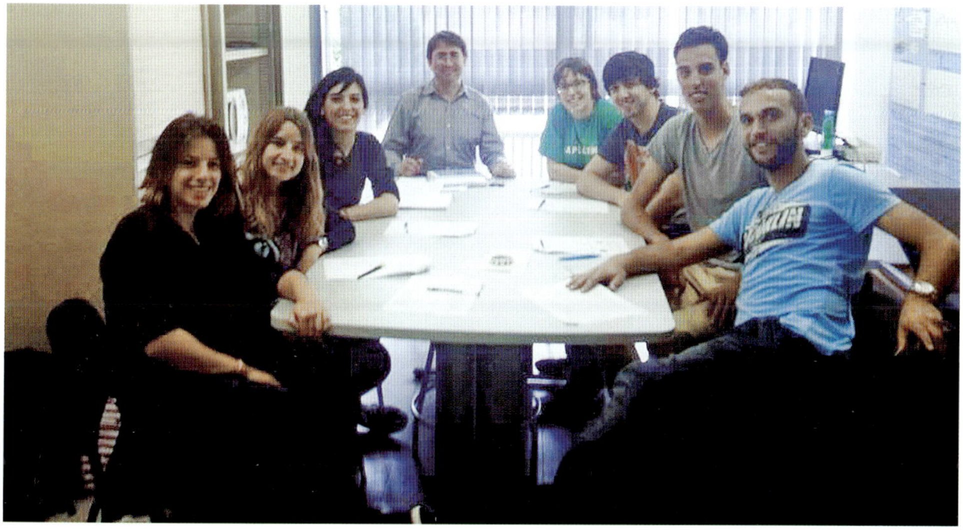

Participants(experiment group) of Study 1

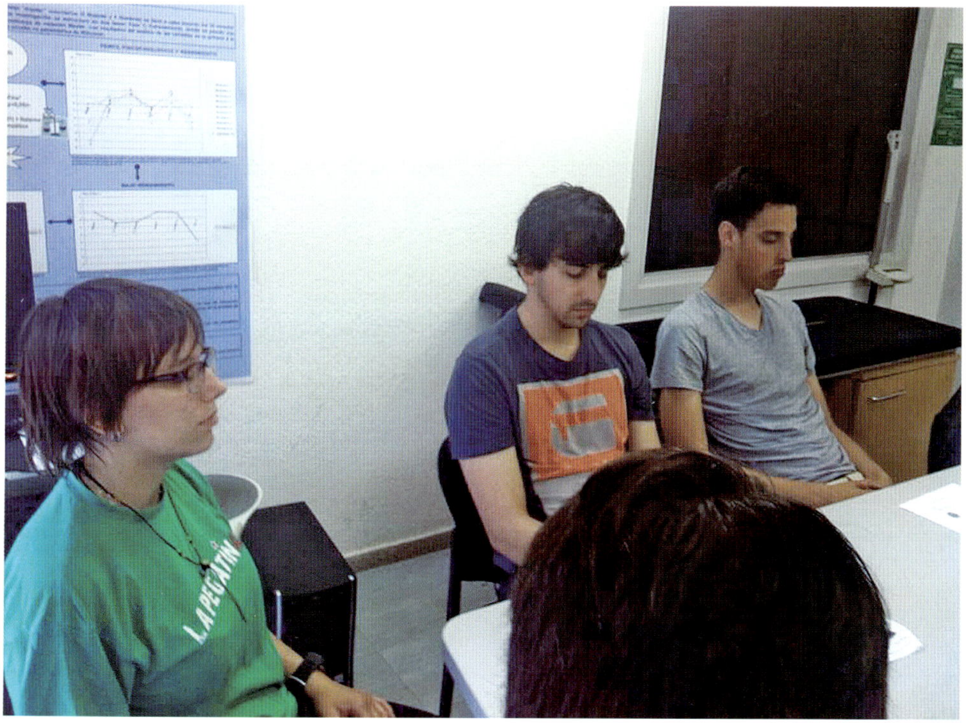

Study 1: Experiment group were testing

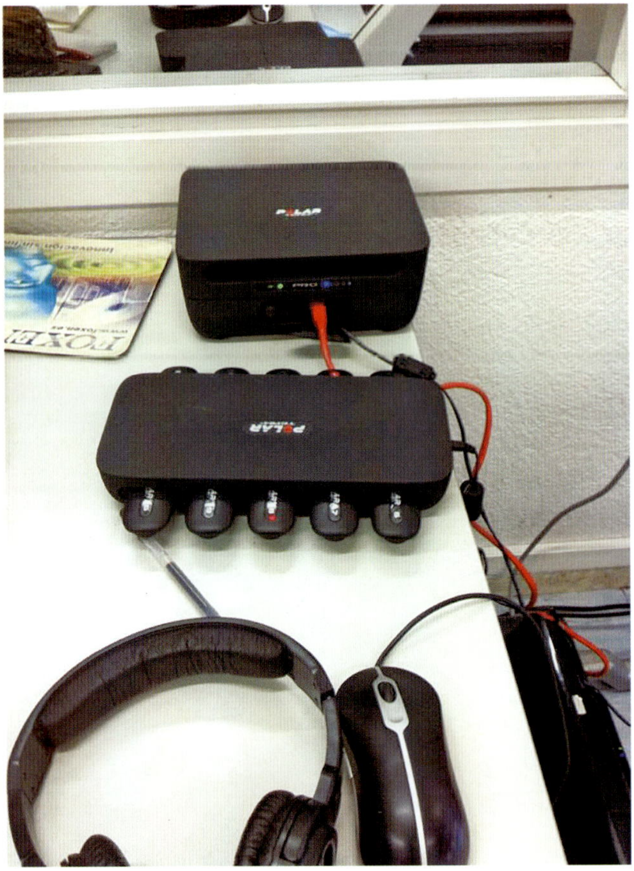

Chest band of HRV

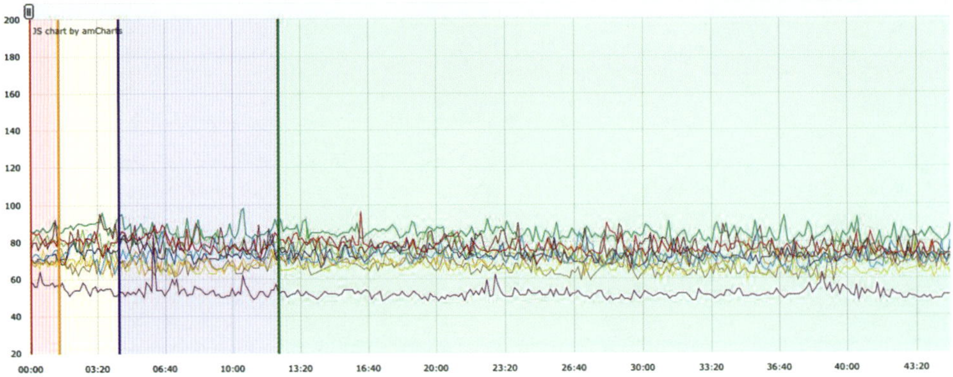

A part of result of Pilot Study 1

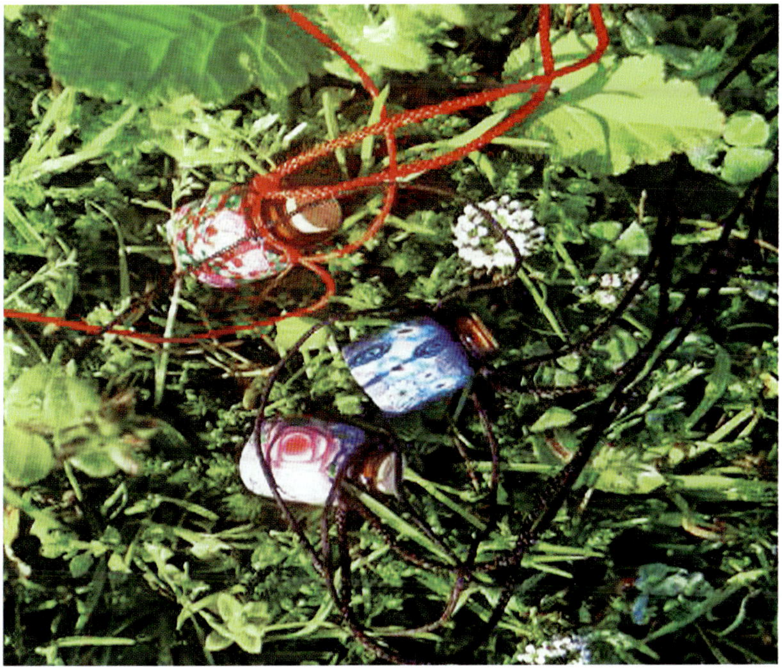

Aroma neckace for participants wear at home

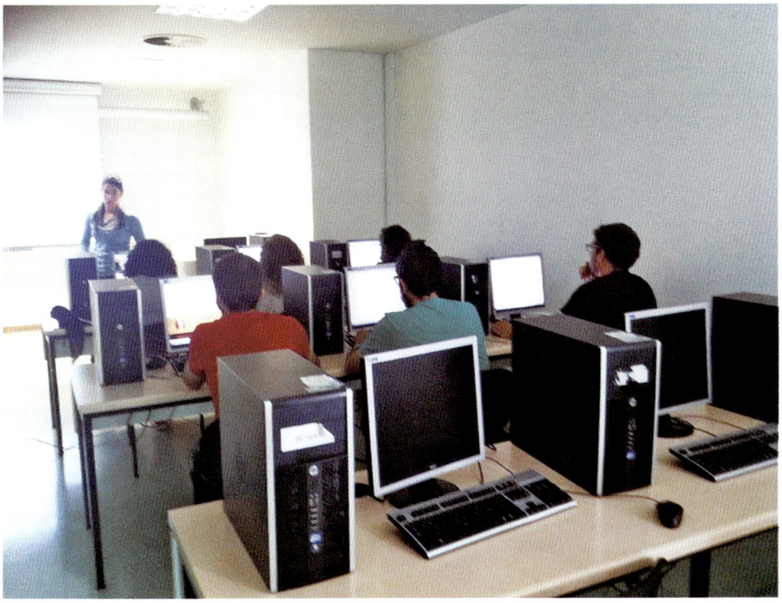

Study 2： Experiment group were testing

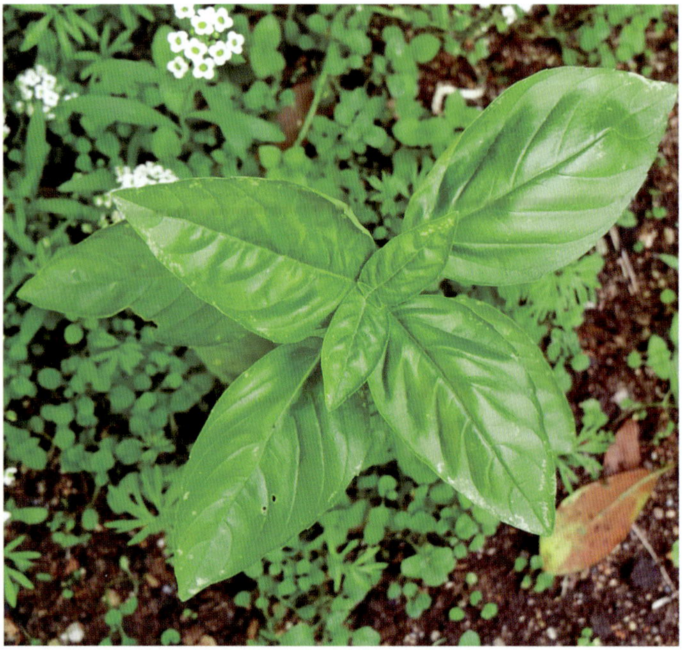

Ocimum basilicum L. (Sweet basil)

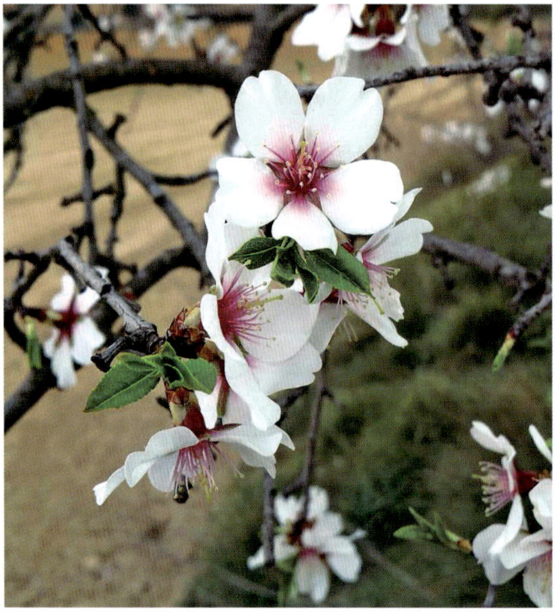

Prunus amygdlus var. *dulcis* (Sweet almond)

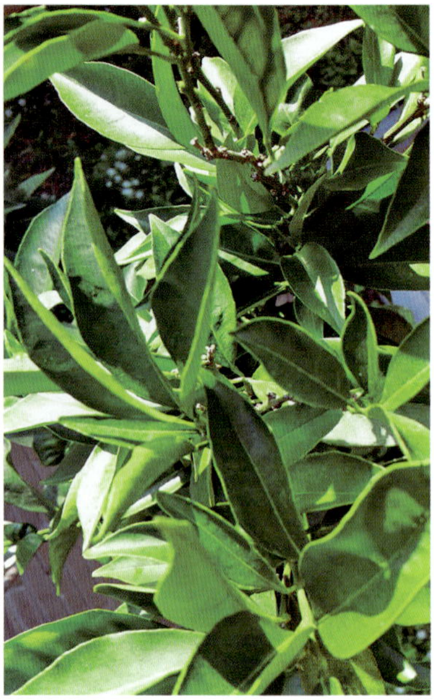

Citrus aurantium bigarade (Petitgrain)

Abbreviations

ANS: autonomic nervous system

AR: aromatherapy

BTv4: bluetooth v4

CAB: *Citrus aurantium bigarade*

CHM: Chinese herbal medicine

CL: *Canarium luzonicum*

CO: *Cananga odorata*

CON: control group

DIF: different

Dur: during

EXP: experiment group

FACE: feeling scale

GLM: general linear model

HF: high frequency

HFnu: HF values expressed in normalized units

HF/LF: the ratio of LF to HF

HR: heart rate

HRV: heart rate variability

LF: low frequency

LFnu: LF values expressed in normalized units

MCS(SF12): mental component summary of SF12

Mean: M

Min: minter

N: number
NS: no significance
OBL: *Ocimum basilicum* L.
OFC: orbitofrontal cortex
PAD: *Prunus amygdalus* var. *dulcis*
PCS(SF12): physical component summary of SF12
POMS: profile of mood states
POST: post intervention(after inhalation period)
PRE: previous period
RMSSD: root mean square of difference of successive RR intervals
RRmean: the mean of RR intervals
SD: standard deviation
SDRR: standard deviation of all RR intervals
SF_ 12v2(or SF12): the 12-item short form health survey
STAI: the state-trait anxiety inventory
STAI_ S: state scale of sate-trait anxiety inventory
STAI_ T: trait scale of state-trait anxiety inventory
TCM: traditional Chinese medicine
VLF: very low frequency
WHO: World Health Organization

Preface

Health psychology has acquired considerable experience and recognition abroad.

The program in health psychology of the Autonomous University of Barcelona (UAB) is a great opportunity for me to study at UAB with the research group "Health, Sport and Lifestyle" coordinated by Dr Lluís Capdevila.

In this book, I could not only study about healthy lifestyle and physical activity, but would also learn many aspects about Catalonia and Spain as ancient and rich historic countries in Europe: The tourism industry, which is highly developed; Spanish people love sports and have a great sense of humor. They are cheerful and enthusiastic; I was so excited that I received the offer from the Health, Sport and Lifestyle research group. If we combine the experience of traditional Chinese medicine treatment and the European empirical research, we shall be open to learn from each other. What a kind of interesting new findings will come to light!

In this book, the focus is about "aroma efficacy in improving negative emotions, attention level, heart rate variability and in performing well in workplace and academic situations, through balancing the autonomic nervous system (ANS)."

The book has two general parts. The first one (theoretical part) is the background of aroma in the main context of traditional Chinese medicine. We will also take a look at the effects of aroma over physical and psychological symptomatology. The second part (empirical part) is dedicated to analyze the aroma efficacy for improving negative emotions, attention level and performance in the workplace and in academic situations.

In order to achieve this general objective, we conducted two main studies (Study 1 and Study 2) with their respective pilot studies (Pilot Study 1 and Pilot Study 2).

1) The Pilot Study 1 is planned to obtain the key information to design the definitive

Study 1, such as the type of essential oil, the number of sessions or the inhalation time duration. The main objective of Study 1 is to analyze the short and long term efficacy of aromatherapy(AR) for reducing anxiety and improving study concentration of university students. For this reason, the Pilot Study 1 was conducted on university students in order to achieve the best results.

2) In the same way, the Pilot Study 2 is planned to obtain the key information to design the final Study 2 carried out with university staff. The main purpose of Study 2 is to analyze the AR efficacy to reduce workplace stress and improve work performance in university administrative workers.

In all studies and pilot studies we will analyze the AR effects over the heart rate variability as a marker of the sympathetic/parasympathetic balance from the ANS. For this purpose, we will use the FitLab Team system (Health & SportLab, Barcelona, Spain).

Contents

List of Tables and Figures

Tables

Figures

Introduction

The general aim of this book is to analyze the aromatherapy(AR) efficacy to reduce negative emotions and increase the attention level and performance in the workplace and in academic situations. Its efficacy will be tested through questionnaires and by checking the balance of the autonomic nervous system(ANS) through HRV analysis. To carry out this general objective, we conducted two main studies. We will analyze the AR effects over the heart rate variability(HRV) as a marker of the sympathetic/parasympathetic balance from the ANS.

The objective for Study 1 is to analyze the AR efficacy for reducing anxiety and improving study concentration in university students. The sample is composed of 12 students(between 18 and 33 years old). We analyze the effects of *Sweet basil* essential oil inhalation at short-time(1 hour) and long-time(1 month). We find that inhalation of *Sweet basil* essential oil reduces the anxiety level and improves cardiac variability(SDRR and RMSSD parameters). AR in a short session or with an aromatic necklace every day during one month produces emotional and HRV changes on participants.

The objective for Study 2 is to analyze the AR efficacy to improve the work performance and reduce the workplace stress. The sample is composed of 42 administrative university workers(age: 42.21, $SD = 7.12$; gender: 10 men and 32 women). All sessions are performed in a university computer classroom. The participants are randomly assigned into an experiment group(EXP) and a control group(CON), and they are invited to participate in a specific session. They are seated in front of computers. During the intervention period, some oil diffusers are launched and worked throughout the session with *Petitgrain* essential oil for EXP sessions and a neutral oil (*Sweet almond*) for CON sessions. At the same time, participants complete a computer task in a specific website typing on their keyboard until they finished it. The single times are different for all participants and are recorded in the website as "Performance time". The EXP performed the website task with the keyboard 2.28 min faster than the CON ($p = 0.05$) and showed better cardiac variability (HF, SDRR and RMSSD parameters). Inhalation of *Petitgrain* essential oil reduces stress and improves performance in the workplace. AR improves the performance time when typing with the keyboard in a simulated computer work session and produces some changes improving HRV.

General conclusions: Our results confirm that aromatherapy (inhaling essential oils) can improve performance in the workplace, can help to manage negative emotions and can increase the attention level in academic and workplace situations. Our results confirm that inhalation of essential oils produces this effect by balancing the sympathetic/parasympathetic system of the autonomic nervous system. HRV analysis is a good marker of this effect. This ANS balance can be explained by a combined action of the main components of *Petitgrain* and *Sweet basil*. Some of them have sedative effects, which can induce changes on the parasympathetic activity, and other have activation effects, which stimulate the sympathetic activity.

The final effect can be an improvement of the mental and emotional condition by a combination of reducing stress level and increasing arousal level of the participants in terms of attentiveness and alertness. We can also explain our results according to TCM. Essential oils can work through a truly holistic therapy, taking into account the mind, the body and the spirit of the person. Essential oils can connect with our bodies and help to find the best way to solve our body's needs. The relaxing effects (parasympathetic activity) can be related to Yin and the activation effects (sympathetic activity) can be related to Yang.

1 The Basic Theory of TCM, Aromatherapy, ANS and HRV

1.1 The Basic Theory of Traditional Chinese Medicine

1.1.1 Background of Traditional Chinese Medicine

Traditional Chinese medicine(TCM) has a history of thousands of years(Hu, Liu, 2012). During the long course of development, it has absorbed much essence from other academic and cultural fields, including traditional Chinese culture, natural sciences, humanities and social studies, making it into a unique system of medicine with extraordinary theory, rich experience and significant therapeutic effect throughout history(Li, Xu, 2011). TCM has contributed a great deal toward the development and prosperity of the Chinese nation. Now it has been disseminated to the other parts of the world and has been extensively studied.

TCM was deeply influenced by ancient Chinese philosophy(Hu, Liu, 2012). It is formed by summarizing the precious experience of understanding life, maintaining health, and fighting diseases accumulated in daily life, production and medical practice. It does not only have systematic theories, but also have abundant of preventive and therapeutic methods to confront diseases. It has also created a visceral manifestation theory and a meridian and collateral theory to explain the structure and physiological function of the human body and the developing laws of disease(Hu, Liu, 2012; Lu, Jia, Cheng, 2004).

1.1.2 Traditional Chinese Medicine Theory of Holism

TCM can be characterized as holism. The theory of TCM holds that the universe is a material integrity and is the result of the mutual opposition and unity between Yin and Yang(Dong, Zhang, 2001). The human body is an organic whole in which the constituent parts are structurally inseparable, functionally coordinated and interactive, and mutually influencing. The theory of TCM emphasizes on the integrity of the human body and the harmony between humans and their social and natural environment, and gives emphasis to the balance between the different systems and organs inside the body. TCM focuses on health maintenance and the treatment of diseases, specially remarking the importance of enhancing the body's resistance to diseases (Zhou, 2008; Dong, Zhang, 2001).

In TCM, illness is regarded as a state of disharmony between the individual and his or her natural and social environments. Accordingly, the aim of TCM is to help people regain a state of harmony. The curative and caring approaches focus not only on treating illnesses but also on counteracting the imbalances, which are the source of illnesses (Hu, Liu, 2012; Dong, Zhang, 2001).

1.1.3 Theory of Yin and Yang

The theory of Yin-Yang is one of the ancient Chinese philosophies that define the reciprocity of matters in the universe. The ancient Chinese thinkers found that every phenomenon has two opposing sides. They adopted Yin-Yang to explain any two matters in the universe that are opposed. Yin and Yang are mutually opposed, but they are also connected. They contend against each other, restrain each other, and mutually repel each other. On the other hand, they are interdependent, they are the root of each other, and mutually generate and promote themselves. Moreover, Yin and Yang are not static; they are constantly growing or diminishing, and even transform into the opposing side under certain conditions. Generally, things that are mobile, exterior, rising, warm and bright pertain to Yang, while things that appear static, interior, descending, cold and dark pertain to Yin. Some examples are male and female, good and bad, top and bottom, left and right, and white and black, but the two contrary elements can be mutually transformed (Hu, Liu, 2012; Dong, Zhang, 2001) (see Figure 1).

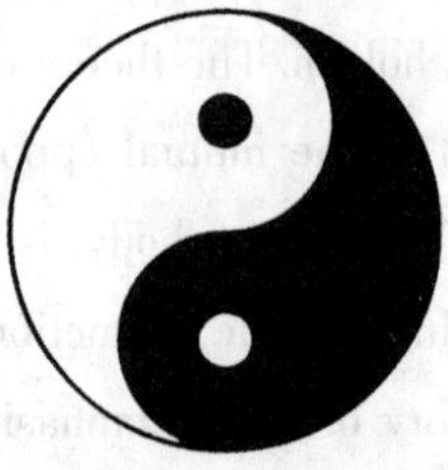

Figure 1 Chinese Yin and Yang symbol

Any two matters in the universe are opposed; Zhou, 2008.

The philosophical theory of Yin and Yang permeates the theoretic system and clinical practice of TCM, which are used to explain the mechanism of balancing the functions of the human body. The theory of TCM holds that maintaining Yin and Yang in balance is the best way of preserving life. The imbalance between Yin and Yang is a source for all diseases. For improving health, TCM applies multiple natural therapeutic methods.

1.1.4 TCM Multiple Natural Therapeutic Methods

TCM therapies are based on the traditional theory of Chinese medicine, through different ways of acting on the human body organs and blood or stimulating the human body acupuncture point, in order to clear the meridians, balance Yin and Yang, Qi and blood to adjust the role of organs. Chinese medicine practitioners can use different treatments to achieve the purpose of treating diseases and health care of the patients.

1.1.4.1 Acupuncture

Acupuncture is a kind of treatment that applies needles, heat, pressure, and other treatments to certain places on the skin, called acupuncture points, to cause a change in the physical functions of the body(Deng, 2001).

The use of acupuncture is a part of TCM. It is a form of alternative medicine involving thin needles being inserted into the body. It is a key component of TCM. And it is a very ancient system, having originated in China over 4,000 years. It is deeply rooted in the Taoist philosophy which recognizes two opposite and complementary energies, Yin and Yang, flowing through the whole of the nature of human beings. Yin and Yang energies are seen as a part of this whole, and flow through the body in a network of pathways called meridians, Yang energy passing down the back of the body and Yin energy up the front of the body. Both are maintained in a subtle and constantly changing balance. While this balance exists, and the energy flows freely, the body is healthy, but if a meridian is blocked at any point, there will be an excess or deficiency of energy, resulting in an illness. By inserting very fine needles at appropriate points on the meridians, the acupuncturist can remove the blockage and restore health (Deng, 2001; Davis, 1992). (see Figure 2)

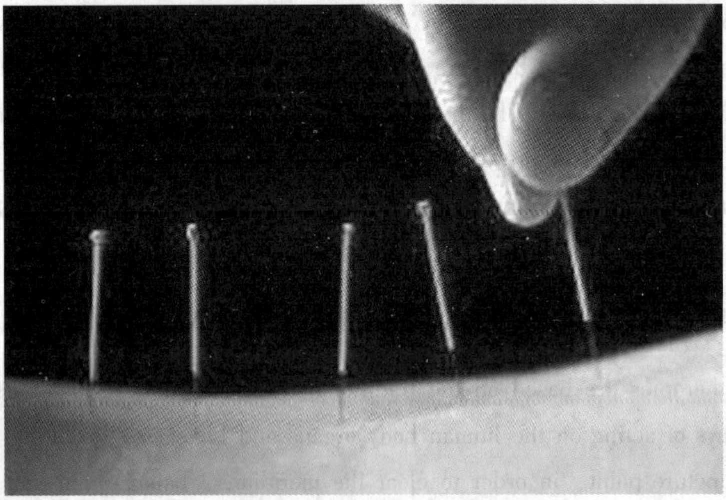

Figure 2 Needles being inserted into a person's skin

Webpage: Southern California Acupuncture, 2016.

1.1.4.2 Tui Na(Meridians Massage and Acupuncture)

The theory of meridians is an essential part of TCM. Meridians refer to the main pathways and collaterals refer to the network of branches. Meridians are longitudinal lines and collaterals are the transverse branches which run all through the body and connect all parts of the body together as shown in Figure 3. Meridians are divided into two groups: twelve regular meridians and eight extraordinary meridians. The twelve regular meridians are connected with the six Zang organs(including pericardium) and the six Fu organs(see Figure 3). The meridians are directly connected with the viscera and each Yin meridian matches a Yang meridian. The twelve regular meridians pertain to either Yin or Yang. One Yin meridian and one Yang meridian are internally and externally related to each other. For instance, the lung and the large intestine are internally and externally related to each other, so constipation can be treated by drugs that increase lung Qi. Thus, an illness can be treated by inserting needles in the acupuncture points located on the right meridians(Zhou, 2008).

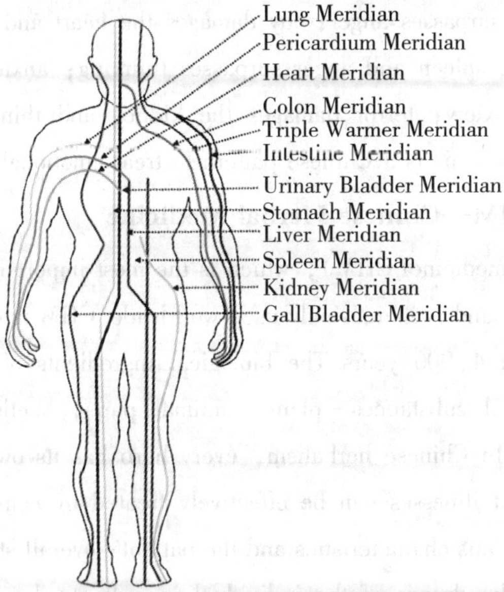

Figure 3 Twelve regular meridians related with the six Zang organs and the six Fu organs

http: //alternativeresourcesdirectory. com/news/what – are – the – meridians. 2019.

1.1.4.3 Negative Emotion Treatment of TCM

In TCM there are seven negative emotions that can cause disease. These seven emotions are normal feelings of human beings, but excessive changes of these emotions may damage the body and cause diseases. The seven negative emotions are joy, anger, anxiety, contemplation, sorrow, terror and fear. Every emotion is controlled by different organs. For example, the heart stores joy. Laughing indicates happiness, but excessive laughing may cause diseases. The heart stores the spirit, excessive laughing disperses the spirit and that is why it is said that excessive joy is harmful to the heart. Excessive anger is related with liver study. The liver is related with the emotions of joy and tenderness, excessive anger will damage liver Qi and result in people losing temper. Excessive anxiety and grief are related with lung and spleen Qi. An excess of anxiety and grief blocks Qi flow, eventually damaging the lung which governs Qi and also damages the spleen due to indigestion. Terror and fear damage kidney Qi. Terror and fear indicate extreme nervousness and timidity, usually caused by deficiency of kidney Qi or blood. Nevertheless, emotions could be influenced by each other: anger damages the liver and sorrow surpasses anger; joy damages the heart and terror surpasses joy; thinking damages the spleen and anger surpasses thinking; anxiety damages the lung and joy surpasses anxiety; terror damages the kidney and thinking surpasses terror (Zhou, 2008). Thus, this is a Chinese pattern to treat emotional disorder.

1.1.4.4 CHM—Chinese Herbal Medicine

Chinese herbal medicine (CHM), which is the most important branch of TCM, is widely used in China and is increasingly used worldwide. CHM is empirically based and has a history of over 4,000 years. The biological ingredients of herbal remedies are extracted from natural substances—plants, animal parts, shells, insects and even stones and minerals. In Chinese herbalism, every herb has its own properties. Chinese herbalists believe that illnesses can be effectively treated by combining herbs, taking into account their various characteristics and the patient's overall status. The composition of the formula and the dosage of the individual ingredients depend on the signs and symptoms of the patient, which is the basic principle of CHM. These formulas can be modified to fit specific individuals more closely (Ruan, Lai, Zhou, 2006).

With the development of society and the constant innovation of science and technology, it has been discovered that the active ingredients of plants can be purified by distillation technology, which opens up a new direction for ancient Chinese medicine therapy. Aromatherapy, which uses a large number of aroma herbs as a basis for any treatment, will become a new area of TCM.

1.2 Aromatherapy

1.2.1 Background of Aromatherapy

Aromatherapy (AR) is an ancient herbal medicine tradition and it was used in some ancient countries, such as Egypt, China and India, thousands of years ago. AR is a kind of natural treatment method utilizing the chemical structure and effects of plants essential oils, which extracted from herbs, roots, leaves, flowers, and other plant parts. They can be used to treat various diseases (Cooke, Ernst, 2000).

AR has significant therapeutic potential because each essential oil has a unique combination of chemical compounds that interact with the body's chemistry and thereby affect specific organs, systems and the body as a whole. For example, some studies have shown that certain essential oils decrease anxiety related behavior and improve some illnesses in humans and animals (Koulivand, Khaleghi Ghadiri, Gorji, 2013).

AR has grown in importance as an area in alternative medicine with proven high efficacy in reducing stress and improving mood disorders (Souto-Maior, de Carvalho, de Morais, *et al.*, 2011). Recently, AR is used by more and more people around the globe, and clinical research into this field is also increasing every year. Some studies reported that inhaling pepper oil induces an increase in adrenaline concentration, while inhaling rose oil decreases the adrenaline level (Haze, Sakai, Gozu, 2002). Some studies have also shown that estragon oil, or grapefruit oil, stimulates effects on the sympathetic and parasympathetic activity. *Ocimum basilicum* L has been traditionally employed as a medicinal herb in the treatment of headaches, coughs, diarrhoea, constipation, warts, and/or kidney malfunction (Joshi, 2014).

1.2.2 Effect of Aromatherapy

Aromatherapy has beneficial effects on our body in two main ways.

1.2.2.1 The Effect of the Physical Symptoms

Some studies show that aromatherapy is useful to reduce physical symptoms, such as pain, cancer, chronic diseases, antibacterial and antiviral diseases. Małachowska, Fendler, Pomykała, *et al.* (2016) discovered that oils reduce autonomous response to pain sensation during self-monitoring of blood glucose among children with diabetes. Shin, Seo, Lee, *et al.* (2016) found that massage with aroma can relief the symptoms in people with cancer. Marchese, Orhan, Daglia, *et al.* (2016) found antibacterial and antifungal activities of thymol. Vitro found antibacterial activity of essential oils against streptococcus pyogenes (Sfeir, Lefrançois, Baudoux, *et al.*, 2013).

1.2.2.2 The Effect of Emotions on Health

Essential oil can be used to change moods, particularly those which are antidepressant and cheering. Virtually any of the uses of essential oils in massage, baths, perfumes and other methods have a beneficial effect on symptoms such as stress, fear, anxiety, withdrawal and depression(Price S, Price L, 1995).

Franco Land and his colleagues found that lavender fleur oil and unscented oil can reduce preoperative anxiety in breast surgery patients(Blanck, Dugan, Kline, *et al.*, 2016). Hosseini and his colleagues(2016) found that inhaling lavender essence could reduce the level of anxiety and blood cortisol in candidates for open-heart surgery. Chamine and Oken(2016) found that aromas have effects on physiological and cognitive function following acute stress.

1.2.3 Essential Oils: The Main Component of Aromatherapy

Essential oils are the principal components of aromatherapy. They are concentrated on volatile compounds formed as secondary metabolites in aromatic plants and characterized by a strong odor(Solgi, Ghorbanpour, 2014). Their biological effects may be the result of the synergistic effect of all the molecules together or only the main molecules found in larger concentrations of these oils. The effectiveness of essential oils is believed to be derived from each of the essential oils with unique chemical components (Bakkali, Averbeck S, Averbeck D, 2008).

Different essential oils depending on the chemical components affect our emotions. For example, on the one hand, terpenes and sesquiterpenes, which are the biggest chemical family in essential oil, could stimulate sympathetic activity. Pinene, myrcene, limonene, caryophyllene and other components were detected in pepper oil, estragon oil, fennel oil and grapefruit oil(Baik, Kim, Lee, *et al.*, 2008). On the other hand, ethers and alcohols induce inhibition of sympathetic activity. Methyl chavicol, anethole, citronellol, geraniol, nerol alcohol, patchouli alcohol and other components were detected in rose oil and patchouli oil(Haze, Sakai, Gozu, 2002). Our study compared two groups of people working on a website and found that the use of *Petitgrain* can make work performance 2.28 min faster. All participants in all groups showed a decrease from PRE to POST in the emotion scales(Huang, Capdevila, 2017).

Pierre Franchomme, a French chemist, invented the structure-effect diagram of essential oils which was a decisive contribution to modern aromatherapy. The structure effect diagram was created to show the impact that the tendency to attract or donate electrons has on the properties of an essential oil component.

The structure effect diagram allows us to connect a physically measurable parameter with the effect of the oils. It provides a tangible model for approaching the scientific concepts of the complicated essential oils chemical composition (Franchomme, Jollois, Penoel, 2001). (see Figure 4)

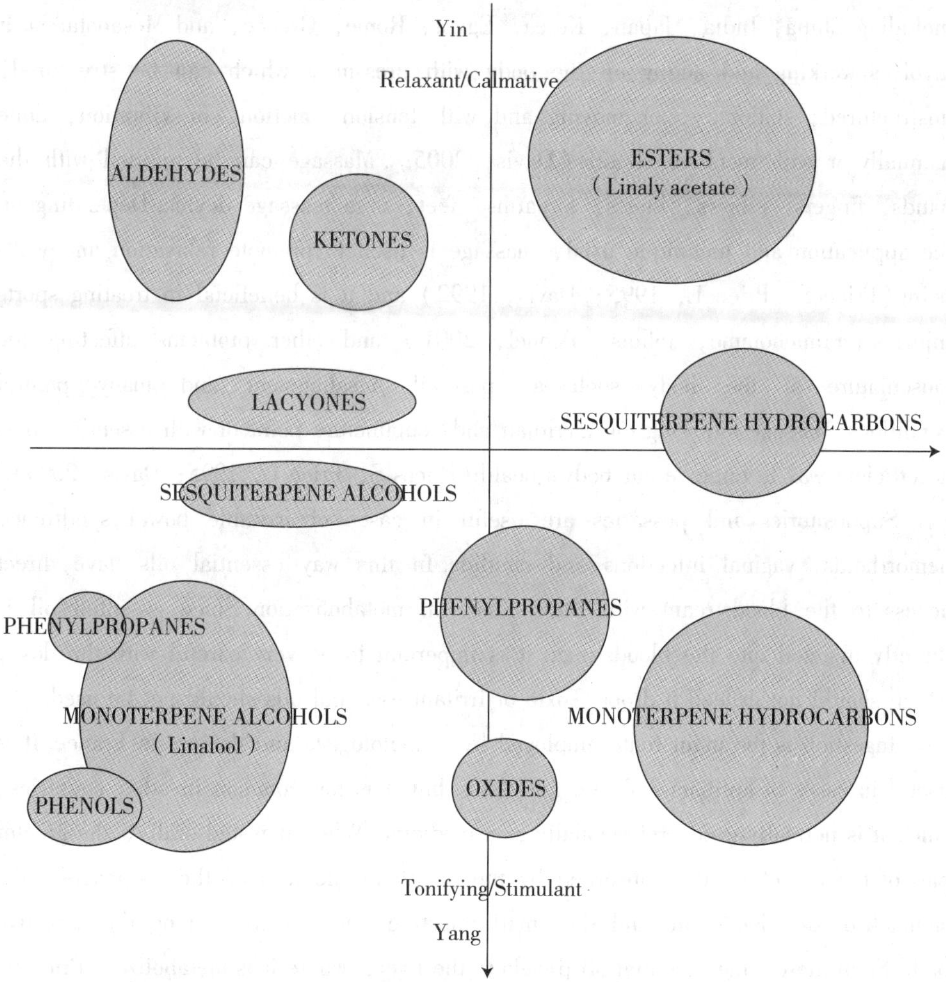

Figure 4 The structure effect diagram of the main components of essential oil

The main components of essential oil can be placed in a coordinate system according to their chemical qualities and their lipophilic or hydrophilic nature.

1.2.4 Pathways of Aromatherapy Working in the Body

The essential oil can be absorbed into the body through four main channels (see Figure 5): 1) through the skin; 2) through anus and vagina suppositories; 3) through the digestive system; 4) through the olfactory system (Price S, Price L, 1995).

Archaeological evidence of massage has been found in many ancient civilizations including China, India, Japan, Korea, Egypt, Rome, Greece, and Mesopotamia. It involves working and acting on the body with pressure, which can be structured, unstructured, stationary, or moving and with tension, motion, or vibration, done manually or with mechanical aids (Davis, 2005). Massage can be applied with the hands, fingers, elbows, knees, forearms, feet, or a massage device. Depending on the application and technique used, massage is used to promote relaxation and well-being (Price S, Price L, 1995; Davis, 1992) and it is beneficial in treating sports injuries (Franchomme, Jollois, Penoel, 2001) and other problems affecting the musculature of the body such as postural misalignment and many painful conditions. Massage following the meridian and acupuncture point or with essential oil is an efficient way to improve our body's health (Prices S, Price L, 1995; Davis, 2005).

Suppositories and pessaries are useful in cases of irritable bowel syndrome, hemorrhoids, vaginal infections and candida. In this way essential oils have direct access to the bloodstream with little effect on metabolization. Since essential oil is directly injected into the bloodstream it is important to be very careful with the dose, which should not exceed 6 drops. Toxic or irritant essential oils should not be used.

Ingestion is the main route employed by primatologists and doctors in France. It is useful in cases of antibacterial and antiviral, but it is not common in other countries, since it is normally used professionally as a medicine. When ingested orally, the greater part of the essential oil is absorbed by the mouth or the throat, the esophagus, the stomach or the duodenum and the small intestine, as it travels along the digestive path. From there, the essential oil travels to the liver, where it is metabolized (Price S, Price L, 1995; Schnaubelt, 1998).

When oils are ingested through the olfactory system, the mechanism of action of inhaled aroma starts with the absorption of volatile molecules through the nasal mucosa

(Stea, Beraudi, de Pasquale, 2104). Then the odor molecules of essential oils are transported to the brain by the olfactory sensory neurons in the nasal cavity. Odor molecules are then transformed into chemical signals, which move towards the olfactory bulb, and possibly to other parts of the limbic system. They stimulate smell memory work, influence memory, thoughts and emotions (Krusemark, Novak, Gitelman, *et al*., 2013) by interacting with the neuropsychological framework to produce psychological effects. Even a small number of molecules inhaled by respiration causes an indirect physical effect by activating the memory or by infiltrating the blood (Krusemark, Novak, Gitelman, *et al.*, 2013; Robins, 1999). (see Figure 5)

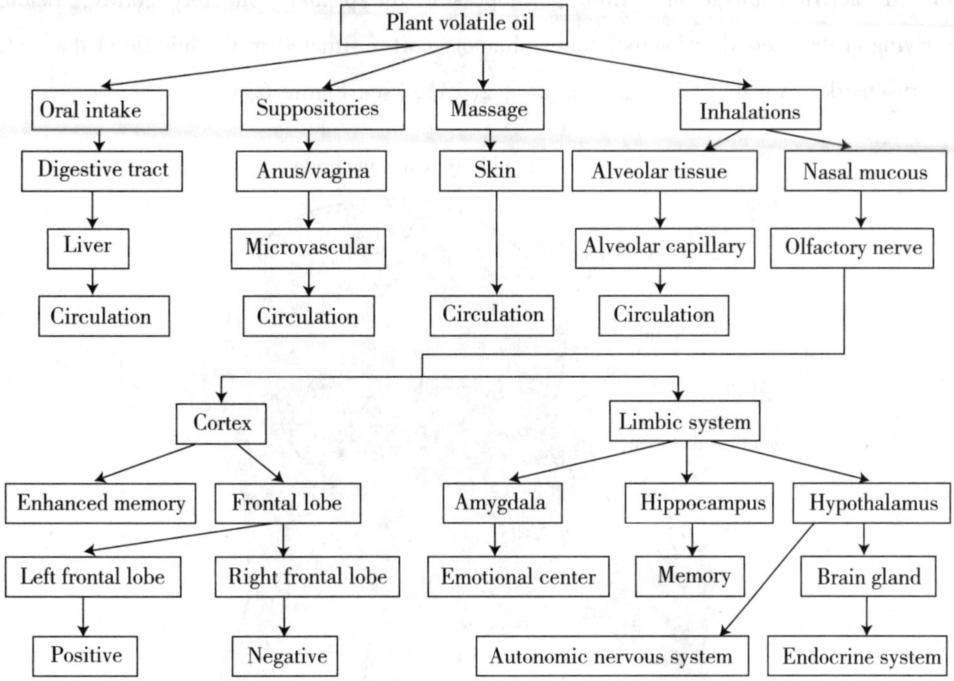

Figure 5 Four main pathways though which essential oils can be introduced into the body

Price S, Price L, 1995. *Aromatherapy for Health Professionals.*

1.3 Two Main Systems of Aroma Inhaling

1.3.1 The Olfactory System

The olfactory sense is phylogenetically the oldest sense. It has a unique intimacy with emotions, unlike other senses. Olfactory neuroanatomy is intertwined, via extensive reciprocal axonal connections, with primary emotion areas including the amygdala, hippocampus, and orbitofrontal cortex (OFC). Olfactory stimulation can directly activate amygdala neurons, by passing the primary olfactory cortex, before arriving at the secondary (association) olfactory cortex situated in the middle of the OFC (Krusemark, Novak, Gitelman, *et al.*, 2013). (see Figure 6)

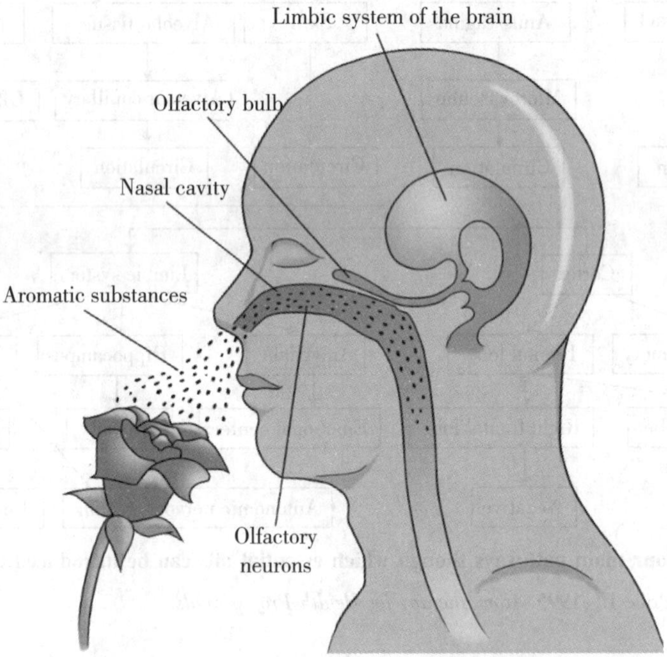

Figure 6 Diagram of the olfactory system

The patch of neurons located at the top of the nose feed into the olfactory bulb which sends signals directly to the brain. Hiawatha olfactory system works, 2011.

The sense of smell plays an important role in the physiological function of the individual because its response is immediate and it is directly extended to the brain; it seems to be related to emotional behavior. The odor molecules of essential oils are transported to the brain by olfactory sensory neurons in the nasal cavity; thus, they stimulate smell-memory work and influence memory, thoughts and emotions (Pierre-Marie L, Gilles G, Jean-Didier V, 2005).

1.3.2 The Autonomic Nervous System

The odor molecules of essential oils are transported to the brain by olfactory sensory neurons located in the nasal cavity and stimulate the autonomic nervous system. Thus, another part of the beneficial effects of aromatherapy is the ANS balance, which manages the sympathetic-parasympathetic interaction (Jänig, 1989).

The autonomic nervous system is a division of the peripheral nervous system that influences the function of internal organs. The autonomic nervous system controls unconscious actions and regulates bodily functions such as heart rate, digestion, respiratory rate, pupillary response, urination, and sexual arousal (Schmidt, Thews, 1989). The autonomic nervous system is composed of two parts, the sympathetic nervous system and the parasympathetic nervous system, which function primarily in opposition to each other. The sympathetic nervous system starts in the spinal cord and travels to a variety of areas of the body. Its function appears to be preparing the body for the kinds of vigorous activities associated with "fight or flight", that is, with running from danger or with preparing for violence, associated with energy mobilization. The parasympathetic nervous system has its roots in the brainstem and in the spinal cord of the lower back. Its function is to bring the body back from the emergency status which the sympathetic nervous system puts into. It is also associated with vegetative and restorative functions (McCorry, 2007). Some studies show that the nervous system has a particularly powerful role to play in our emotional life (Boeree, 2002; Shin, Liberzon, 2010).

1.4 Heart Rate Variability

Heart rate variability refers to the variation in the time interval between consecutive heartbeats (the RR interval). HRV analysis is a valid and reliable method to check the ANS balance and it can be used to evaluate the AR effectivity. (Chang, Shen, 2011; Cervantes, Rodas, Capdevila, 2009)

Finally, it should also be taken into account that there is a trend to use uncommon essential oils, often derived from wild plants which have a tendency to produce numerous cultivars with different chemical compositions. The different chemo types have often not been tested toxicologically, and further problems could possibly derive from this in an uncontrolled market.

2　Approaches, Objectives and Hypotheses

2.1 Approaches

In the introduction part of this book we found that numerous studies have shown that negative emotions are associated with bad health, such as cardiovascular disease, diabetes, cancer, musculoskeletal problems, or alcohol dependence, and even with mortality. In fact, negative emotions constitute the most potent risk factor for suicide. Depression, stress and anxiety are the most prevalent negative emotions related with health problems in the world that result in an enormous burden on the health care system. The World Health Organization (WHO) has envisaged that negative emotions related with chronic psychiatric disorders will become the second leading cause of premature death or disability worldwide by the year 2020(Reddy, 2010).

In the European Union, 350 million work days are lost because of negative emotions related problems, resulting in an overall cost of at least 20 billion euros every year. This problem has been noted by the European Commission(Taelman, Vandeput, Vlemincx, *et al.*, 2011).

Increasingly, experts call for the implementation of human health promotion programmed. In particular, people who suffer from negative emotion problems should be identified at an early stage so that preventive action can be taken. Thus, many depression, stress and anxiety reduction related methods have been investigated and various approaches have been involved in negative emotions management. Aromatherapy is one of these approaches thanks to its easy implementation and effectiveness(Chang, Shen, 2011).

At present, aromatherapy is used by more and more people around the globe, and clinical research into this field is also increasing every year. This discipline has grown in importance as an area in alternative medicine with proven high efficacy in improving negative emotions and mood disorders. But there are some important questions to answer about the action mechanisms of aromatherapy and about the scientific evidence of its effects.

2.2 Objectives

The general aim of this book is to analyze the aromatherapy efficacy to reduce negative emotions and increase the attention level and performance in the workplace and in academic situations. Its efficacy will be tested through questionnaires and by checking the balance of the autonomic nervous system through HRV analysis.

To carry out this goal objective, we conducted two main studies (Study 1 and Study 2) with their respective pilot studies (Pilot Study 1 and Pilot Study 2). The specific objectives for each study are:

2.2.1 Objectives for Study 1

1) Analyzing the AR efficacy for reducing anxiety and improving study concentration in university students.

2) Analyzing the long-term effect of different AR oils on negative emotions and attention level in academic situations.

3) Analyzing the AR acute effects during one-hour inhalation.

2.2.2 Objectives for Study 2

1) Analyzing the AR efficacy to reduce workplace stress and improve work performance.

2) Analyzing the effect of different AR oils on stress and performance in the workplace.

2.2.3 Objective for Both Studies

The focus of both studies are about 1) "aroma efficacy in improving negative emotions, attention level, HRV and in performing well in workplace and academic situations, through balancing the autonomic nervous system"; 2) analyzing the AR effects on the HRV as a marker of the sympathetic/parasympathetic balance from the ANS.

2.3 Hypotheses

1) Inhalation of *Ylang ylang* or *Sweet basil* essential oils can reduce academic anxiety and improve study concentration in university students (Study 1).

2) Inhalation of *Elemi* or *Petitgrain* essential oils can reduce stress and improve performance in the workplace (Study 2).

3) Inhalation of essential oils has its deepest acute effects at 20 – 25 min after starting inhaling (Study 1).

4) AR has short-term efficacy (1 hour) and long-term efficacy (1 month) to reduce negative emotions (both studies).

5) Inhalation of essential oils can reduce negative emotions by balancing the sympathetic/parasympathetic system of the autonomic nervous system, and HRV analysis can be a marker of this effect.

6) Inhalation of *Ylang ylang*, *Sweet basil*, *Elemi* or *Petitgrain* will increase the HRV and reduce the questionnaire scores of negative emotions.

3 General Materials and Methods

3.1 Questionnaires

Wc will resume the cognitive instruments we used in all studies.

1) A global "Feeling Scale" asking for "How do you feel today." Participants had to choose one value from 0 ("very bad") to 10 ("very good") scales. The Feeling Scale will be used to assess the participants feeling state before and after sessions.

2) A short version of profile of mood states (POMS) (Shacham, 1983). The POMS consists of 15 items, three for each subscale (*tension*, *depression*, *hostility*, *vigor* and *fatigue*). The *tension* scale indicates that the higher the score, the more nervous the participant is; the *depression* scale indicates that the higher the score, the more sadness the participant feels; the *hostility* scale indicates that the higher the score, the more hostility towards others the subject feels; the *vigor* scale is a positive scale and suggests that the higher the score, the more energy the participant has; the *fatigue* scale indicates that the higher the score, the more fatigue the participant feels. All these five scales contain three items that are scored according to a scale from 0 ("nothing") to 10 ("very much"). The POMS will be used to assess mood states before and after the sessions.

3) The state-trait anxiety inventory (STAI) (Spielberger, 2010). This instrument is divided into two scales, each having 20 questions. The first subscale measures state anxiety (STAI_ S) and the second measures trait anxiety (STAI_ T). The participants were asked to rate the intensity of each symptom on a scale from 0 ("not at all") to 3 ("very much"), resulting in scores ranging from 0 to 60. The scale indicates that the higher the score, the more anxiety state or trait the participant has. STAI_ T scale will be administered immediately prior to the first session and immediately after the last session. STAI_ S scale will be used to assess anxiety state before and after the sessions.

4) SF_ 12v2 (SF12) Health Survey is a 12-item short form of SF_ 36v2 global instrument (Schmidt, Thews, 1989). The 12 answers are based on a Likert scale from 2 to 6 answer options, which permit to obtain two global scores: physical component summary [PCS (SF12)] and mental component summary [MCS (SF12)]. SF_ 12v2 will be administered immediately prior to the first intervention and immediately after the last

intervention.

3.2 Heart Rate Variability Analysis: Instruments and Procedures

We perform HRV analysis in all studies and sessions. Participants' session ratings of continuous heart rate (RR or beat to beat cardiac intervals) are collected and analyze with FitLab Team system (Health & Sport Lab, Barcelona, Spain). It consists of an application that runs in a mobile device (iPad, Apple) connect via bluetooth v4 (BTv4) with several cardiac chest bands (H7 model) to obtain RR intervals, and connect via wireless with a remote server (Health & Sport Lab). The system permits to perform synchronize recordings of all participants in each session and check at real time the quality of the data. Typically, participants are asked to remain at rest in the same position, without speaking or making any movements, and heart rate variability data is registered continuously following a natural breathing. FitLab Team system uses Polar technology which validate for detecting RR intervals at rest (Parrado, Garcia, Romas, *et al.*, 2010). The digitized signal is filtered, in accordance with common standards, and processed by the FitLab software to obtain and filter the RR series, and calculate several HRV parameters. For the time domain analysis, these HRV parameters are: the mean of RR intervals (RRmean); the standard deviation of all RR intervals (SDRR); and the root mean square of difference of successive RR intervals (RMSSD). For frequency domain analysis, all RR series are resampled at 3 Hz using a cubic spline prior to the HRV analysis. The power spectrum of the resampled time series is estimated using the Fast Fourier Transform after removing the mean of the time series and multiplying the time series by a Hann window. The HRV frequency parameters are: the power of the very low frequency (VLF) band, which is estimated by integrating the power spectrum for frequencies lower than 0.04 Hz; the power of the low frequency (LF) band, computed in the band 0.04 – 0.15 Hz; and the power of the high frequency (HF) band, computed in the band 0.15 – 0.4 Hz. Additional calculations included the ratio of LF to HF, LF and HF values expressed in normalized units (LFnu and HFnu). The calculation of these indices is consistent with the recommendations of the Task Force of the European Society of Cardiology (ESC) and the North American Society of Pacing and Electrophysiology (NASPE) (Moreno, Ramos-Castro, Rodas, 2015).

To control these variables, which can influence heart rate variability, in all sessions, participants are asked not to consume any food of beverages containing alcohol or caffeine after the evening of the day preceding the session. They are also asked not to do vigorous physical activity during 24 hours before being test.

3.3 Aroma Instruments and Procedures

3.3.1 Aroma Instruments

Essential oils (100% pure):

1) *Ocimum basilicum* L. Abbreviation = OBL. English name: *Sweet basil.*

2) *Citrus aurantium bigarade.* Abbreviation = CAB. English name: *Petitgrain.*

3) *Canarium luzonicum.* Abbreviation = CL. English name: *Elemi.*

4) *Cananga odorata.* Abbreviation = CO. English name: *Ylang ylang.*

All essential oils were diluted to 2% before being used in our studies.

Vegetable oil (100% pure):

Prunus amygdalus var. *dulcis.* Abbreviation = PAD. English name: *Sweet almond.*

Sweet almond is a kind of vegetable oil with natural smell. It was diluted to 2% before being used in our studies.

In our text we will use the English oil names. In tables and figures we will use abbreviations of Latin names.

3.3.2 Aroma Intervention Procedures

Aroma intervention was conducted once a week, a total of 4 – 6 weeks in the lab, in the work site or at home, depending on the study. HRV parameters were recorded during lab sessions.

1) An ultrasonic lonizer aroma diffuser was used for aroma evaporation in the lab.

2) Aroma necklace was used for aroma evaporation at home or in the work site.

Detailed experimental procedures were as follows.

1) Basic aroma interventions were conducted on workdays in the morning. Smoking and drinking alcohol or coffee was forbidden during six hours before the aromatherapy session.

2) Lab sessions: Participants were asked to rest for 5 minutes before performing any task. Then, a 40 – 90 min aroma inhalation took place.

3) Aroma inhaled at home: Participants conducted 3 hours of aroma inhalation at home wearing the aroma necklace.

4 Study for Determining Whether Aroma Reduces Anxiety and Improves Attention

4.1 Objective

The aim is to conduct a pilot study for determining the procedures and characteristics of aroma methods, based on the meridian system, to reduce anxiety and to improve attention control in a university environment. This information will be useful to conduct the definitive study later.

4.2 Sample

The participants were five postgraduate students, five participants completed two initial lab sessions, four completed the third session and three completed the all sessions. (aged 24, 26 and 33; gender: 1 male and 2 females) . All participants agreed to collaborate voluntarily and provided informed consent before participating in the pilot study. They met the following inclusion criteria: 1) no clinical diagnosis of autonomic dysfunction; 2) no clinical diagnosis of respiratory, cardiovascular, endocrine or systemic disorder; 3) no problems with their olfactory function; 4) none of the participants had been clinically diagnosed with diabetes mellitus, hypertension, hyperlipidemia, asthma, cardiovascular disorders, or any other endocrine or systemic disorders that could affect the autonomic nervous system.

4.3 Instruments

For this pilot study we used the FitLab Team system(see Chapter 3 Section 2) to analyze HRV and the questionnaire STAI_ S, POMS, the Feeling Scale, SF_ 12v2 and STAI_ T(see Chapter 3 Section 1). We also used lifestyle questionnaire interviews as qualitative research instruments to collect data about the lifestyle behaviors of participants during the days that they used the aroma.

Participants interviews took place during the lab sessions. Themes explored included symptoms, effects, management of the aroma, willingness, sleeping habits and lifestyle behaviors (see items in Table 1) . Interviews were digitally transcribed and analyzed. This information helped to identify aromatherapy specific situations and challenges for a more effective management(Chien, Cheng, Liu, 2012).

Table 1 Interview of lifestyle questions to collect data about the lifestyle behavior of participants during the days that they used aroma at home

Code	Question	Result
1	How was your sleep and dream pattern?	Good/Average/Poor
2	Have you eaten regularly?	Yes/No
3	How was your stool?	Good/Average/Poor
4	What time did you usually smell the essential oil?	Morning/Afternoon/Night
5	How was your learning attention when smelling the oil?	Good/Average/Poor
6	How was your learning attention during this week?	Good/Average/Poor
7	Do you like the aroma?	Yes/No
8	Do you like this way to use essential oil?	Yes/No
9	Did you feel any change on your emotions after smelling the oil?	Yes/No
10	Are your emotions more positive or more negative after smelling the oil?	Positive/Negative

4.4 Procedure

4.4.1 General Procedure for All Sessions

We did not inform participants about which fragrance or essential oil we were going to use for the study. We conducted this pilot study through 4 sessions in different weeks and conditions(see Table 2).

Participants went to the lab in 4 group sessions distributed in different weeks. All sessions were performed in the morning between 9:00 and 11:00 in a quiet lab environment. In all the sessions the ambient temperature was between 22℃ and 25℃.

In general, the intervention in each session consisted in a 20 min self-massage with a specific essential oil on a specific acupuncture point and a 45 min aroma inhalation of a specific essential oil. All participants performed a total of 4 sessions in 4 weeks.

Table 2 Characteristics of the 4 sessions conducted in the Pilot Study 1 with participants

Session	Participants	Time	Place	Oil	Use way
Session 1	3	90min	Lab	CO	Smell and massage
Session 2	3	90min	Lab	CO	Smell
Session 3	3	90min	Lab	OBL	Smell and massage
Session 4	3	90min	Lab	OBL	Smell

CO: *Ylang ylang*. OBL: *Sweet basil.*

1) When the group of participants arrived at the lab they were asked to rest in a sitting position in front of a circular table, like in their classroom. In general, they followed the steps of Figure 7.

2) Participants were required to fill out the PRE questionnaires. (STAI_ S, POMS, SF_ 12v2 and the Feeling Scale).

3) Participants were asked to wear the cardiac chest band (connected via bluetooth to an iPad with FitLab software) and sit at ease around the table.

4) HRV_ PRE (before aroma inhale) was recorded for 5 minutes with the participants at this rest situation: sitting, opening eyes, putting hands on their knees, doing no activity, breathing naturally and speaking nothing.

5) A specific aroma was scattered in the environment and participants could be required to self-massage an acupuncture point of their hands in Session 1 and 3 (see Figure 8). At the same time, they were inhaling the aroma and the HRV was recorded during a minimum of 45 minutes.

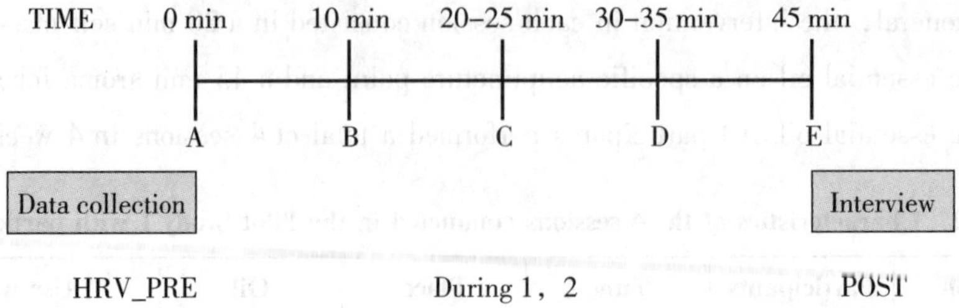

Figure 7 General experimental procedure and data collection for Pilot Study 1

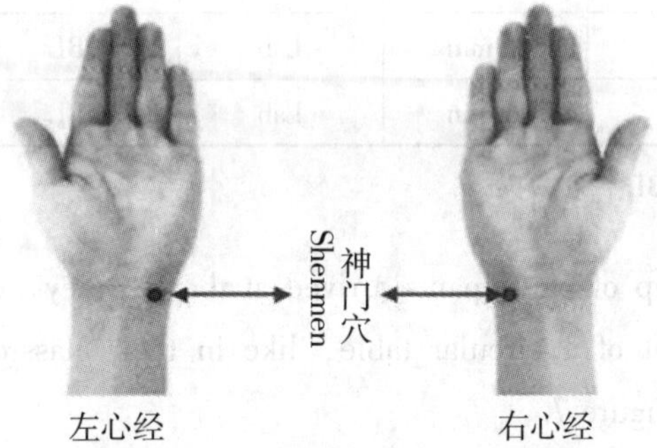

Figure 8 TCM acupuncture points of "*Shenmen*"

淘中医之宝，2016.

6) Participants were required to perform a 5 min HRV posttest (sitting, opening eyes, putting hands on their knees, doing no activity, breathing naturally and speaking nothing).

7) Participants were asked to fill out the POST questionnaires (STAI_ S, POMS and the Feeling Scale).

8) A short interview was performed for participants who used the aroma at home. (except for Session 1)

STEPS:

(1) Before: STAI and POMS questionnaires.

Participants were asked to (2) wear the cardiac chest band; (3) PRE—5 min HRV pretest; (4) A) starting the oil inhalation and/or hand massage, B) massaging the other hand, C) (During 1) finishing massage and starting the 5 min HRV test, D) (During 2) 5 min HRV test, E) finishing inhalation and (5) starting POST—5 min HRV posttest.

(6) After: STAI and POMS. (7) Short interview.

PRE: 0 - 5 min PRE.

During 1: 20 - 25 min.

During 2: period between 30 - 35 min.

POST: 5 min POST.

4.4.2 Specific Procedure for Session 1

The participants followed the general procedure and step (1) to (3) explained above. At the beginning of the fourth step, *Ylang ylang* aroma was scattered in the room through the diffusers (see Chapter 3 Section 2) for all the remaining session. This allowed a proper aroma inhalation throughout the complete lab room. In the fourth step, participants were also required to massage themselves on the left hand on the acupuncture point of "*Shenmen*" for 10 min (see Figure 8). This massage was performed clockwise with the right hand. Then, a clockwise massage with the left hand on the acupuncture point of "*Shenmen*" on the right hand was performed another 10 minutes. After this time the participants stopped the massage and sat at rest situation until completing the remaining session steps.

At the end of the session, participants were asked to wear a necklace (see Chapter 3 Section 3) for 7 days and inhale the *Ylang ylang* oil during 3 hours per day at home. The specific instructions were: "You have to inhale the aroma for 3 hours at home by opening the aroma necklace whenever you prefer and you have to write down how you feel during the inhalation."

4.4.3 Specific Procedure for Session 2

The participants followed the general procedure and step (1) to (3) explained previously. At the beginning of the fourth step, *Ylang ylang* oil was scattered in the room through the diffusers (see Chapter 3 Section 3) for all the remaining session. This allowed a proper aroma inhalation throughout the complete lab room. Then, participants followed the general procedure and step (5) to (7) explained previously.

During the week between Session 1 and Session 2, all the participants used a necklace at home to inhale the *Ylang ylang* oil whenever they preferred, at least 3 hours a day for a period of 7 days in total.

4.4.4 Specific Procedure for Session 3

The participants followed the general procedure and step (1) to (3) explained previously. At the beginning of the fourth step, *Sweet basil* oil was scattered in the room through the diffusers (see Chapter 3 Section 3) for all the remaining session. This allowed a proper aroma inhalation throughout the complete lab room. In the fourth step, participants were also required to massage themselves on the acupuncture point of "*Shenmen*" on their left hand for a period of 10 minutes (see Figure 8). The massage was performed clockwise with their right hand. Then, a clockwise massage with their left hand on the acupuncture point of "*Shenmen*" of their right hand was performed another 10 minutes. After this time the participants stopped the massage and sat at rest until completing the remaining session steps.

During the week between Session 2 and Session 3, all the participants used a necklace at home to inhale the *Sweet basil* oil whenever they preferred, at least 3 hours a day during a period of 7 days in total.

4.4.5 Specific Procedure for Session 4

The participants followed the general procedure and step (1) to (3) explained above. At the beginning of the fourth step, *Sweet basil* oil was scattered in the room through the diffusers (see Chapter 3 Section 3) for all the remaining session. This allowed a proper aroma inhalation throughout the complete lab room. Then, participants followed the general procedure and step (5) to (7) explained above.

During the week between Session 3 and 4, all participants used their necklace at home to inhale the *Sweet basil* oil whenever they preferred, at least 3 hours a day during a period of 7 days in total.

4.5 Results

In this part, we will present the most relevant results of this pilot study for obtaining the key information to design the definitive study (Study 1: Chapter 5).

Among the 5 initial participants, 3 participants completed all sessions of the pilot study. The initial participants constituted a heterogenic sample: postgraduate students of different ages (24, 26, 33 years old), 1 male and 2 females. All participants showed sufficient compliance with the HRV control variables (not taking medicines, doing low level of physical activity and not drinking coffee before HRV analysis).

In order to check aromatherapy effects over arousal and concentration, we analyzed the effects of inhaling *Sweet basil* and *Ylang ylang* oils on HRV through Sessions 1, 2, 3 and 4.

In order to confirm if inhalation aroma is useful and have different effect depending on the period, we analyzed HRV parameters in four periods for every session.

1) PRE: 5 min with the participants at rest before starting aroma inhalation.

2) During 1: 5 min at 20 – 25 min after starting aroma inhalation.

3) During 2: 5 min at 30 – 35 min after starting aroma inhalation.

4) POST: 5 min with the participants at rest at the end of the session.

HRV parameters were calculated in four 5 min periods for each session: PRE, 20 – 25 min (During 1); 30 – 35 min (During 2) and POST.

Table 3 shows the HRV parameters at baseline (PRE, before inhalation), during the inhalation at 20 – 25 min and at 30 – 35 min, and after the inhalation POST, for each of the 4 sessions (2 sessions for CO and 2 for OBL). The differences were at baseline (PRE), 20 – 25 min, 30 – 35 min and POST for the following HRV spectral parameters: LF, such that *Sweet basil* showed a larger decrease between PRE and 20 – 25 min than *Ylang ylang* did, and *Ylang ylang* showed a larger LF increase between 20 – 25 min and POST than *Sweet basil* did; RMSSD, such that *Sweet basil* showed a larger RMSSD decrease between 20 – 25 min and POST than *Ylang ylang* did, and *Ylang ylang* showed an RMSSD increase at this stage (see Table 3). We observe a tendency to significance for HFnu and LFnu. There were no significant differences between the two aromas for LF/HF and RRmean.

Table 3 Means and SD of HRV parameters for the 3 participants and for each of the 4 sessions(2 sessions for CO and 2 for OBL)

Aroma	Session	RRmean/ms	SDRR/ms	RMSSD/ms	LF/ms²	HF/ms²	LF/HF	LFnu/%	HFnu/%
OBL	Session 1								
	PRE	983.04±181.26	148.73±52.62	143.06±45.40	86.37±106.83	117.71±100.62	1.40±0.86	63.64±13.31	46.35±13.31
	Dur 1	1060.61±76.85	109.09±12.71	119.40±6.28	35.38±7.95	42.32±11.21	0.90±0.46	45.83±11.73	54.15±11.73
	Dur 2	1024.59±70.57	82.16±11.25	97.38±37.14	16.88±6.06	36.08±24.17	0.81±0.79	38.64±22.35	61.35±22.35
	POST	116.18±4.13	116.86±13.93	103.53±19.28	9.55±4.70	39.87±15.08	1.43±1.36	50.37±27.70	50.27±28.12
	Session 2								
	PRE	927.29±249.28	131.76±36.43	94.47±22.48	37.48±9.77	40.74±20.68	1.29±1.17	49.74±19.86	50.25±19.85
	Dur 1	862.53±369.85	98.35±6.32	97.63±26.75	26.73±1.91	38.53±10.46	0.72±0.21	41.65±6.85	58.33±6.84
	Dur 2	1029.97±146.52	94.59±11.20	91.70±44.01	23.61±12.30	28.33±19.15	2.25±3.16	48.38±32.36	51.61±32.36
	POST	1007.38±132.79	137.13±21.66	96.09±34.17	22.88±8.68	46.92±22.32	3.40±2.62	67.25±28.72	33.73±28.72
CO	Session 3								
	PRE	1023.65±146.44	122.45±45.53	102.27±54.20	45.07±27.15	47.43±36.19	1.36±0.82	54.71±13.14	45.27±13.14
	Dur 1	1027.12±106.61	125.05±56.31	112.11±67.73	45.22±41.04	42.30±30.76	2.77±1.22	71.26±10.66	28.72±10.67
	Dur 2	993.21±151.53	127.34±47.48	105.49±61.34	32.83±24.82	43.44±37.09	3.07±2.12	68.31±21.15	31.67±21.14
	POST	1022.43±114.52	123.63±52.44	106.60±52.65	34.66±22.46	40.87±29.02	2.55±2.01	66.07±17.79	34.58±18.26
	Session 4								
	PRE	1073.96±146.43	87.11±3.44	78.74±18.66	22.09±6.87	22.90±7.30	1.08±0.56	49.16±15.56	50.83±15.56
	Dur 1	1066.30±228.45	135.80±53.94	116.57±19.45	47.14±65.08	37.78±13.95	2.12±1.81	55.03±34.77	44.95±34.77
	Dur 2	1069.49±162.14	133.93±44.56	126.79±29.51	27.23±5.19	39.49±13.13	1.95±1.75	58.89±18.24	41.09±18.25
	POST	1116.67±199.09	115.02±28.02	78.74±18.66	45.42±33.64	40.04±16.89	1.58±1.43	51.52±30.29	49.13±30.69

HRV: heart rate variability. RRmean: the mean of RR intervals. SDRR: standard deviation of all RR intervals. RMSSD: root mean square of difference of successive RR intervals. LF: low frequency. HF: high frequency. LF/HF: the ratio of LF to HF. LFnu: LF values expressed in normalized units. HFnu: HF values expressed in normalized units. OBL: *Sweet basil*. CO: *Ylang ylang*. PRE: previous period. POST: post intervention(after inhalation period).

Figure 9 and Figure 10 show a change of LFnu and RMSSD at 20 – 25 min(During 1) after starting the *Sweet basil* inhalation from baseline (PRE). The values of these parameters increased at 20 – 25 min from PRE. Figure 11 shows a change of LFnu at

20 - 25 min (During 1) after starting the *Ylang ylang* inhalation from baseline (PRE). The values of these parameters increased at 20 - 25 min from PRE. In both cases, the peaks were at 20 - 25 min.

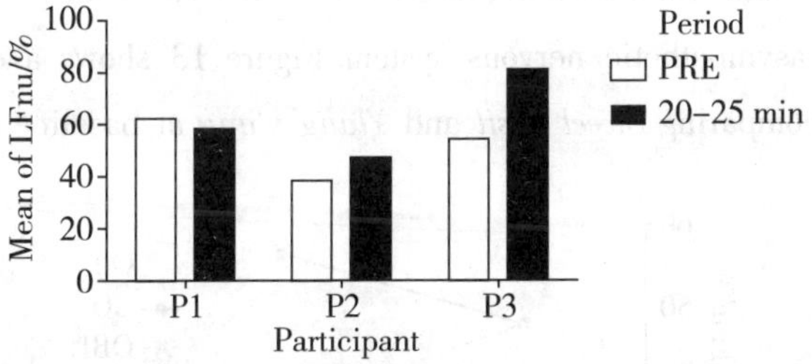

Figure 9 Mean of LFnu parameter for the 3 participants and 2 sessions after the inhalation of *Sweet basil* (comparing the periods PRE and 20 - 25min; Session 1 and 2)

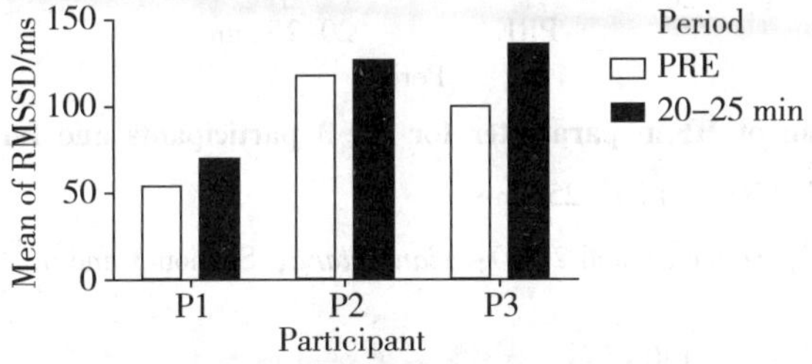

Figure 10 Mean of RMSSD parameter for the 3 participants and 2 sessions after the inhalation of *Sweet basil* (comparing the periods PRE and 20 - 25min; Session 1 and 2)

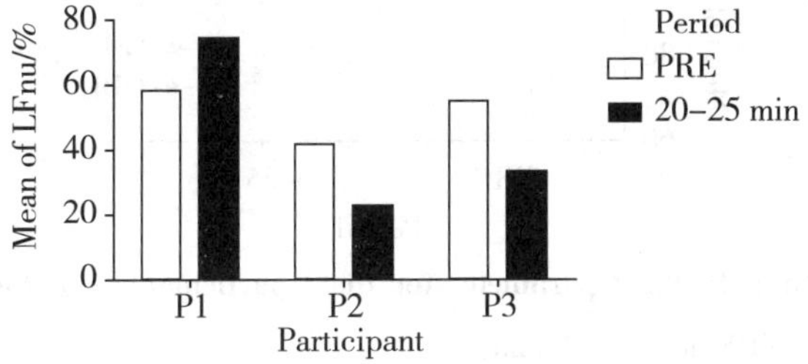

Figure 11 Mean of LFnu parameter for the 3 participants and 2 sessions after the inhalation of *Ylang ylang* (comparing the periods PRE and 20 - 25min; Session 3 and 4)

Figure 12 and 13 show HFnu and RMSSD at baseline (PRE) and During 1 (20 - 25 min) comparing the 2 essential oils, *Sweet basil* in Session 1 and 2, and *Ylang ylang* in Session 3 and 4. Figure 12 shows a different inhalation effect on HFnu comparing *Sweet basil* and *Ylang ylang* at baseline and 20 - 25 min. For HFnu parameters, we observed a bigger increase at 20 - 25 min when inhaling *Ylang ylang* oil, and a deeper decrease at 20 - 25 min when inhaling *Sweet basil* oil. That means inhaling *Ylang ylang* oil more affect parasympathetic nervous system. Figure 13 shows a different inhalation effect on RMSSD comparing *Sweet basil* and *Ylang ylang* at baseline and 20 - 25 min.

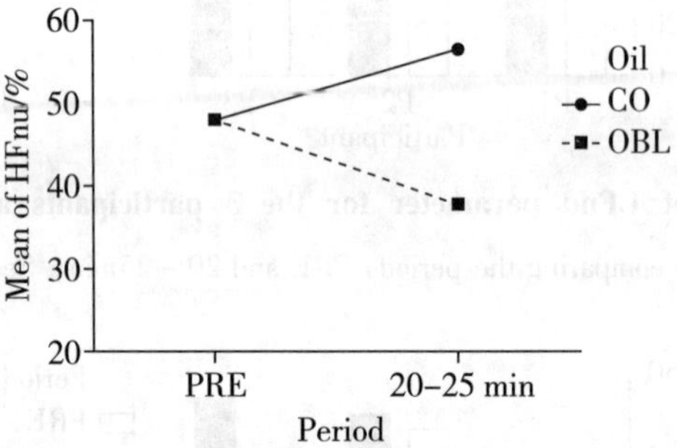

Figure 12 Mean of HFnu parameter for the 3 participants and for the 2 essential oils (comparing the periods PRE and 20 - 25min)

OBL: *Sweet basil*; Session 1 and 2. CO: *Ylang ylang*; Session 3 and 4.

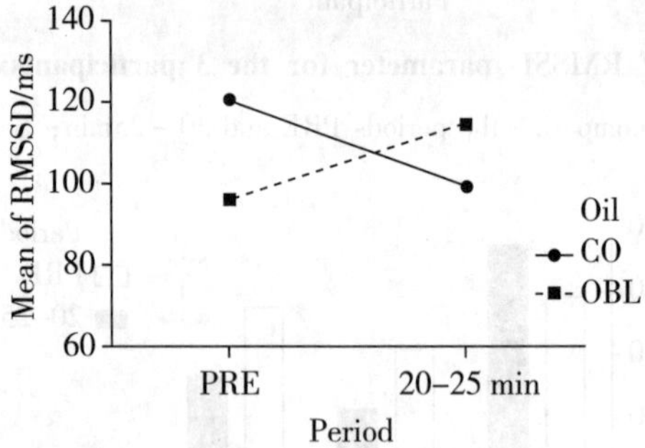

Figure 13 Mean of RMSSD parameter for the 3 participants and for the 2 essential oils (comparing the periods PRE and 20 - 25min)

OBL: *Sweet basil*; Session 1 and 2. CO: *Ylang ylang*; Session 3 and 4.

We found that RMSSD increased when inhaling *Sweet basil* (OBL) and decreased when inhaling *Ylang ylang* (CO) at 20 - 25 min comparing PRE. That means inhaling *Ylang ylang* the participants are tonifying and stimulant and inhaling *Sweet basil* the participants are relaxant and calmative at that time. Inhaling *Sweet basil* oil, the participants trend to increase their heart rate variability.

4.6 Discussion

The pilot study tried to set the best conditions to evaluate the effects on HRV of *Ylang ylang* and *Sweet basil* oil through acupuncture point massage, essential oil inhalation or the combination of both techniques. We wanted to know if HRV analysis is a useful method to explain the effect of aroma inhalation on human sympathetic/parasympathetic autonomic balance. We employed time and frequency domains to calculate HRV parameters as used in previous studies.

We studied the combination of reducing the anxiety level and increasing the attention and cognitive function with the aid of HRV analysis among university students.

In this study, we have chosen very common situations in which students usually find themselves during a normal study day at university, such as typing on their computers, reading, writing, etc.

The data shows a greater improve on HFnu and RMSSD of HRV parameters on *Sweet basil* and *Ylang ylang* oil stimulations at 20 – 25 min after starting inhalation.

However, when we compared the data, we found that when inhaling the *Sweet basil* oil, RMSSD increased more than inhaling *Ylang ylang* oil at 20 – 25 min. When inhaling *Ylang ylang* oil, HFnu increased more than inhaling *Sweet basil* oil at 20 – 25 min. When inhaling *Sweet basil* oil, the participants' attention and cognitive function increased and RMSSD increased too, which means that the participants were more relaxed and calm.

We also analyzed the cognitive levels of anxiety and mood state as stress symptoms in our study, but we did not find significant differences among the participants.

We found a clinically meaningful change in HRV parameter related to anxiety. Participants felt less anxious in the presence of *Sweet basil* and *Ylang ylang* oil. In other words, the level of anxiety of the participants was lower after inhaling *Sweet basil* and *Ylang ylang* oil.

We also found that the highest HRV parameter changed at 20 – 25 min after inhaling the aroma. In this sense, Kuroda, *et al.* found that HF power increased more significantly at 21 min after a 6 min olfactory stimulation of linalool (Matsumoto, Asakura, Hayashi, 2013). In the same line, we found changes at 20 – 25 min after starting the smelling period. This finding is also consistent with the agitation results previously described.

The data showed that aromatherapy would be effective in promoting parasympathetic activation and heart rate. Therefore, aromatherapy may be useful to provide quality of study cognitive function and to reduce study anxiety of university students. Similar to previous research reporting beneficial changes in cognition after aroma exposure, Eguchi and her colleagues found that aromas have protective effects by reducing anxiety. This is another evidence that some aromas may protect cognitive functions. (Eguchi, Funakubo, Tomooka, *et al.*, 2016)

This change could be explained by the combined action of aroma main components (Franchomme, Jollois, Penoel, 2001). On the one hand, some of these components have sedative effects, such as esters, sesquiterpene hydrocarbons, linalyl acetate and linalool, which could induce changes on the parasympathetic activity(Haze, Sakai and Gozu, 2002). On the other hand, methyl chavicol is another component in aroma that could have some activation effects by stimulating the sympathetic activity, as shown in Figure 14. The main components of *Sweet basil* oil are methyl chavicol(7%) and linalool (40% – 50%) and phenols(6%). (see Figure 14) The main components of *Ylang ylang* oil is esters(5%), sesquiterpene hydrocarbons(33% – 38%), phenylpropanes (15%) and monoterpene alcohols 30% (Franchomme, Jollois, Penoel, 2001). (see Figure 15) The main chemical composition of *Sweet basil* and *Ylang ylang* oil is different, and the effects for the participants are different. The result in this study is generally consistent with previous studies, which showed that the sympathetic and parasympathetic nervous systems activity of the participants was stronger after inhaling aromas.

Overall, our study agrees with the importance of aroma as a way to improve attention control in a university environment and reduce study anxiety of university students.

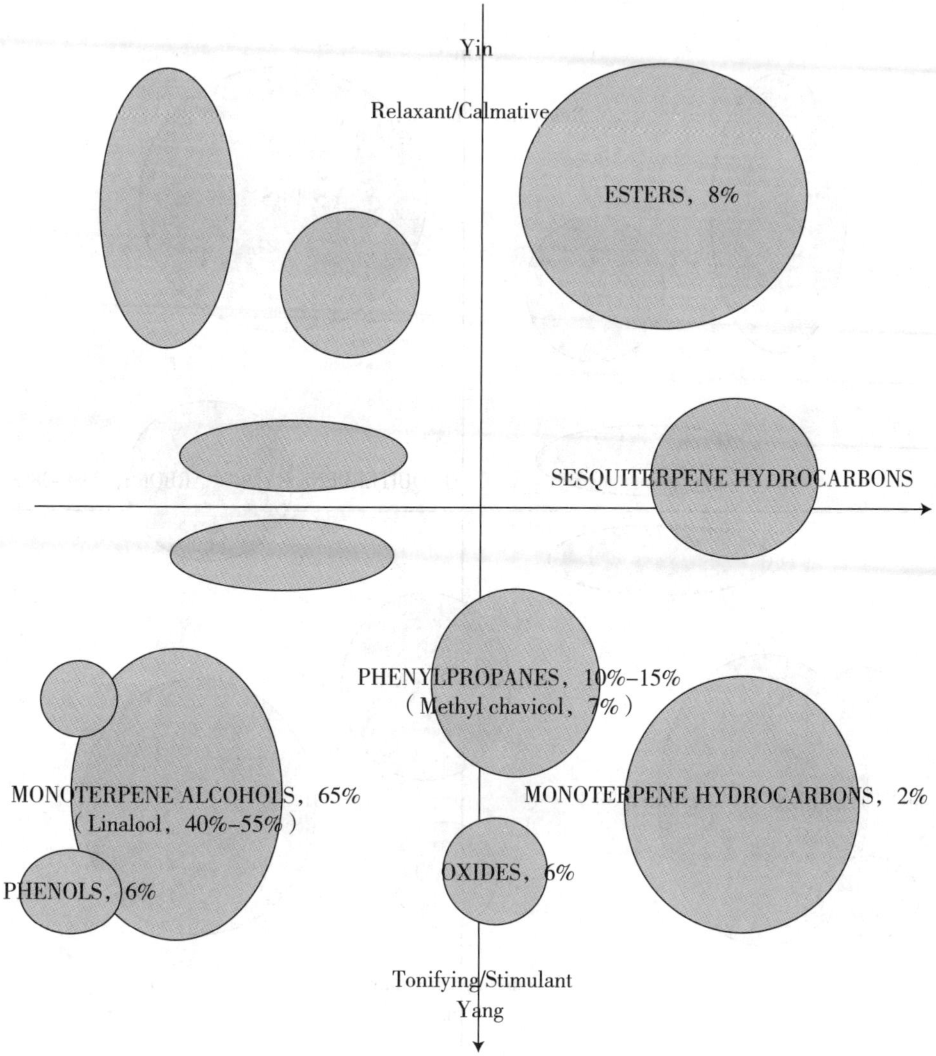

Figure 14 *Ocimum basilicum* main chemical compositions

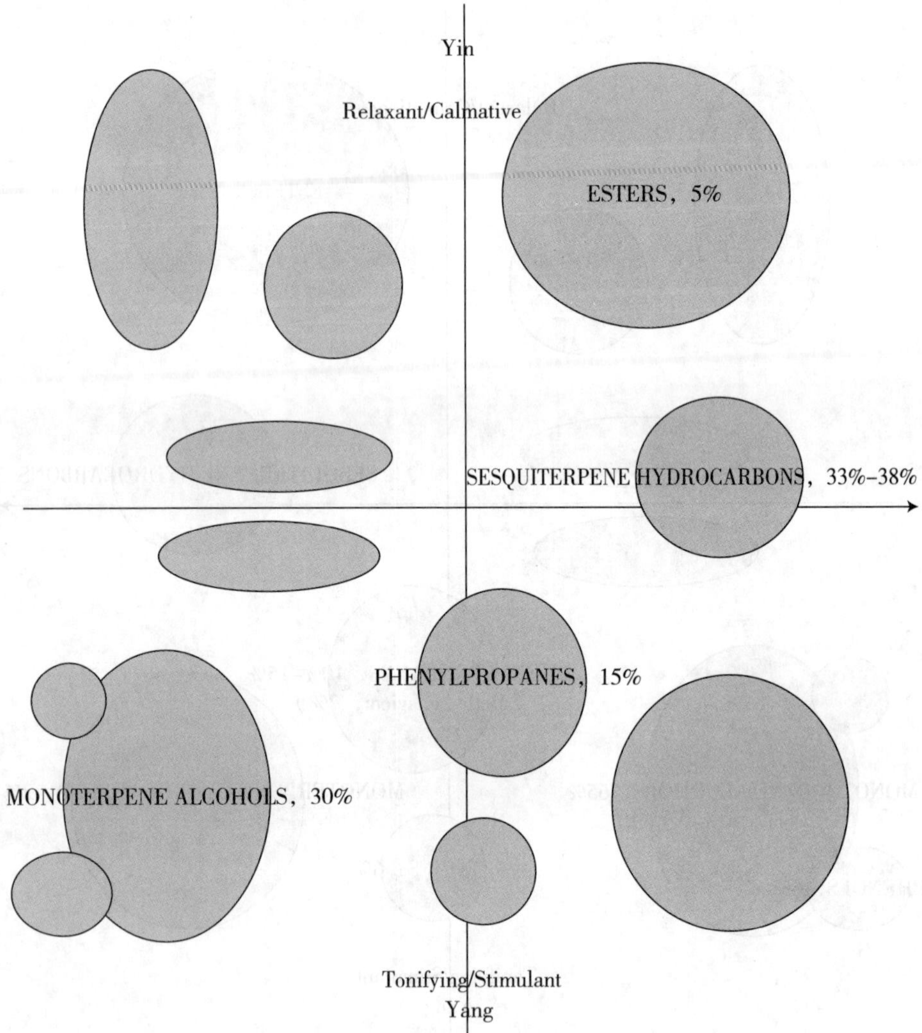

Figure 15 *Cananga odorata* main chemical compositions

We also analyzed the use of a massage on an acupuncture point with aroma inhalation together, but it is not clear what kind of intervention works among the participants. We analyzed the data in Session 1 and 2, with *Sweet basil* inhalation, and Session 3 and 4, with *Ylang ylang* inhalation. We found that when we use the two methods in the same session, it was not clear which method gave better results.

In this pilot study we have found that both *Sweet basil* and *Ylang ylang* oil supposed a clinically meaningful change. But *Sweet basil* oil increased students' attention and cognitive function more than *Ylang ylang* oil. Therefore, we used *Sweet basil* oil in Study 1 (Chapter 5).

4.7 Conclusion

Our study confirms that the use of aroma inhalation of *Sweet basil* and *Ylang ylang* oil together with a massage on an acupuncture point can reduce the anxiety level and increase the attention and cognitive function of university students. We have compared the result of using *Sweet basil* oil and *Ylang ylang* oil. We found that *Ylang ylang* oil have sedative effects, which could induce changes on the parasympathetic activity and reduce anxiety at the same time. *Sweet basil* oil could have some activation effects by stimulating the sympathetic activity and reduce anxiety at the same time. Both oils have shown changes when we compared the PRE and POST parameters aroma. However, our study focuses on increasing the attention and cognitive function and reducing the anxiety level of university students. Thus, this pilot study has ensured that it will be better to use *Sweet basil* oil in Study 1.

We have done a qualitative research in our study. After the interview, we found that participants felt uncomfortable when massaging an acupuncture point by themselves, but in our data the effects of acupuncture massage was not significant. Therefore, in our future study, we will not use acupuncture massage.

5 Aroma Reduces Anxiety and Improves Attention Control in University Students

5.1 Objective

The aim of the study is to determine if aromatherapy reduces anxiety and improves study concentration of university students.

5.2 Sample

The initial sample was composed of 21 healthy undergraduate students (age: between 18 and 33; gender: 7 males and 14 females). They were recruited from a university school through publicity and registration. First, all participants completed a standardized health questionnaire in a previous collective session in order to accomplish the following inclusion criteria: 1) age between 18 and 33; 2) no clinical diagnosis of autonomic dysfunction; 3) no clinical diagnosis of respiratory, cardiovascular, endocrine or systemic disorder; 4) no problems with olfactory function. All participants consented to collaborate voluntarily and provided informed consent before participating in the study. The ethics committee of the university approved the study in advance.

A randomized controlled trial was used. The participants were recruited from some university students through an email advertisement. Twelve participants completed all sessions of the study, seven in the experimental group and five in the control group. We did not inform participants about what kind of fragrance we would use for the sessions.

5.3 Instruments

For this study we used the FitLab Team system (see Chapter 3 Section 2) to analyze HRV and the questionnaire STAI_ S, POMS, SF12 and the Feeling Scale (see Chapter 3 Section 1). The participants inhaled the essential oils through two diffusers that allowed a proper smelling throughout the room. We used two kinds of oils, one for each group: 1) Experiment group (EXP) inhaled *Sweet basil* (OBL). 100% pure OBL was used and diluted to 2%. The predominant constituents were linalool (40% – 55%), methyl chavicol (7%) and phenol 6%. 2) Control group (CON) inhaled *Sweet almond* oil (*Prunus amygdalus* var. *dulcis*. abbreviation: PAD. American, Production batch: YA637, Neroly Company Limited, Hong Kong). The predominant constituents were palmitoleic acid(60% -68%), linoleic acid(17% -30%) and palmitic acid(6% -8%). PAD is a vegetable oil and has a neutral effect for smelling.

5.4 Procedure

In order to distinguish the specific effects of aromatherapy reducing anxiety and improving quality of study in university students, we conducted this study with 4 sessions for all participants. Each group attended 3 sessions separately in different days (CON and EXP had to inhale different oils scattered in the lab) and a final session on the exam day. Thus, Session 1 to Session 3 were performed in different days for each group between 9: 30 and 11: 00 in a lab situation. Session 4 was performed between 9: 30 and 11: 00 in two separate classrooms (one for each group) during a postgraduate exam at the same time. We controlled the ambient temperature for all sessions between 22℃ and 25℃. The intervention consists on inhaling essential oil for EXP and vegetable oil for CON during 45 min in Session 1 to 3, and during 90 min in Session 4 (see Table 4).

Table 4 Sessions characteristics for Study 1

Session	Participants	Time	Place	Oil	Use way	Homework	Group
Session 1	7	45min	Lab	OBL	Smell	No	EXP
Session 1	5	45min	Lab	PAD	Smell	No	CON
Session 2	7	45min	Lab	OBL	Smell	Yes	EXP
Session 2	5	45min	Lab	PAD	Smell	Yes	CON
Session 3	7	45min	Lab	OBL	Smell	Yes	EXP
Session 3	5	45min	Lab	PAD	Smell	Yes	CON
Session 4	12	90min	Classroom 1	OBL	Smell	No	EXP
			Classroom 2	PAD			CON

5.4.1 Procedure for Session 1 to 3

In Session 1 to 3, which took place in the lab, the participants were asked to breathe normally during around 60 minutes in the lab while sitting around a shared table. They were asked not to do any vigorous physical activity, just do the normal things that they usually do in the university classroom, such as reading, writing or using a computer. Two oil diffusers were scattered all over the room. All participants were asked not to consume any food or beverages containing alcohol or caffeine after the evening of the day preceding the experiment. They were also asked not to do vigorous physical activity during 24 hours before the lab sessions. Firstly, participants were required to fill out the PRE questionnaires (STAI_ S, POMS and the Feeling Scale). Secondly, participants were asked to wear the cardiac chest bands (bluetooth connected) and rest in a sitting position at the table. After that, HRV _ PRE was recorded for 5 min with the participants at this rest situation: sitting, opening eyes, putting hands on their knees, doing no activity, breathing naturally and speaking nothing. In the fourth place, the participants inhaled *Sweet basil* (EXP) or *Sweet almond* (CON) thanks to the aroma launched by the diffusers. It allowed a proper smelling throughout the room around 45 min and HRV was recorded during all this time. Then, a 5 min HRV posttest was recorded (sitting, opening eyes, putting hands on their knees, doing no activity, breathing naturally and speaking nothing). After that, participants were asked to fill out the POST questionnaires (STAI _ S, POMS and the Feeling Scale). Then, participants were asked to take an aroma necklace (*Sweet basil/Sweet almond*) for inhaling *Sweet basil* (EXP) or *Sweet almond* (CON) during 3 hours per day at home. (Session 1) Then, an interview about participants' feelings related to the aroma at home was performed (Session 2 and 3).

5.4.2 Procedure for Session 2

The general procedure for Session 2 was the same as Session 1 and 3, but we performed HRV analysis continuously all along the session. We calculated the HRV parameters before starting inhalation (baseline) and after starting it in periods of 5 min at 20 – 25 min and 30 – 35 min.

5.4.3 Procedure for Session 4

The participants arrived at the lab in the morning on the exam day. The first 3 steps were the same with the previous sessions. But in the fourth step, participants went to a different classroom for CON and EXP, mixed with other students who also had the same exam and wore the cardiac chest bands. In Classroom 1, EXP participants inhaled *Sweet basil* aroma from the diffusers which allowed a proper smelling all over the classroom. In Classroom 2, CON participants inhaled *Sweet almond* aroma under the same conditions as the EXP. HRV was recorded during all the exam time(about 90 min). After finishing their exam, the participants were required to perform the HRV posttest in the same exam classroom (sitting, opening eyes, putting hands on their knees, doing no activity, breathing naturally and speaking nothing). Finally, participants were asked to fill out the POST questionnaires(STAI_ S, POMS and the Feeling Scale).

5.5 Results

5.5.1 Results for Study 1(4 Sessions)

Seven participants completed the study in the EXP and five in the CON. Nine of the 21 initial participants did not complete the study because they could not attend 50% of the lab sessions. Table 5 shows the defining characteristics of participants. There were no significant differences between the two groups in terms of gender, age, physical activity level, anxiety trait (STAI_ T), health perception (SF12) and academic performance. Likewise, no significant differences between the two groups were found in terms of HRV control variables, such as taking medicines, doing physical activity and drinking coffee. Thus, these results ensure that there were equal characteristics among the participants in both groups.

Table 5 Participants characteristics for Study 1(gender, age, initial questionnaires and physical activity level for the two groups)

Variable	CON(N = 5)	EXP(N = 7)	p value
Gender			NS
Females	4	4	
Males	1	3	
Age(years)	24. 00 ± 4. 69	22. 29 ± 1. 25	NS
Exam result	8. 04 ± 0. 97	7. 24 ± 1. 09	NS
STAI_ T	18. 67 ± 3. 80	16. 57 ± 10. 40	NS
STAI_ S	24. 40 ± 7. 77	14. 58 ± 6. 18	NS
PCS(SF12)	49. 48 ± 10. 07	52. 56 ± 3. 18	NS
MCS(SF12)	35. 71 ± 8. 83	41. 95 ± 6. 35	NS
FACE	6. 00 ± 1. 63	7. 57 ± 1. 13	NS
Tension(POMS)	5. 44 ± 2. 81	2. 28 ± 1. 56	NS
Hostility(POMS)	0. 78 ± 0. 50	0. 23 ± 0. 49	NS
Fatigue(POMS)	3. 88 ± 1. 63	2. 66 ± 1. 40	NS
Depression(POMS)	1. 83 ± 1. 16	0. 67 ± 0. 96	NS
Vigor(POMS)	5. 77 ± 1. 31	6. 33 ± 1. 66	NS
POMS total	5. 54 ± 0. 66	4. 43 ± 0. 53	NS
Physical activity			NS
No active	80% (4)	71. 4% (5)	
Active	20% (1)	28. 6% (2)	

CON: control group. EXP: experimental group. STAI_ T: trait scale of the state-trait anxiety inventory. STAI_ S: state scale of the state-trait anxiety inventory. PCS (SF12): physical component summary of SF12. MCS(SF12): mental component summary of SF12. POMS: profile of mood states.

5.5.2 Long Term Results: Aromatherapy Effects Through 4 Sessions

In this part we will present the results to explain the AR effects through the 4 sessions of the study. Table 6 and Figure 16 and 17 show SF12 scores(Means and SD) in the 4 sessions for both groups(EXP and CON). General linear model(GLM) analysis which compared the evolution through the 4 sessions, showed significant differences between both groups. Therefore, on the one hand, EXP increases PCS in Session 3 and 4, while CON decreases PCS through the sessions($F_{(3)}$ =4.37; p =0.01)(see Figure 16). On the other hand, CON increases MCS in Session 3 and 4, meanwhile EXP maintains the same MCS scores through the sessions($F_{(3)}$ =3.44; p =0.03)(see Figure 17).

In the case of the physical component summary(PCS) of SF12, one-way ANOVA for each session shows that the only difference(with tendency to significance) between groups is in Session 3. In this session, EXP shows a bigger PCS change than CON ($F_{(9,1)}$ =3.66; p =0.08). There are no significant differences between the sessions for all other SF12 scores including MCS component.

Table 6 SF12 scores(Means and SD) in the 4 sessions of Study 1(for both groups)

Quest	Group	Session 1	Session 2	Session 3	Session 4
PCS(SF12)	CON	56.80 ±6.92	56.50 ±2.17	54.62 ±3.05	53.96 ±4.83
	EXP	56.64 ±5.27	53.87 ±5.82	58.62 ±3.74 *	57.63 ±4.47
MCS(SF12)	CON	43.17 ±8.85	48.86 ±7.44	54.62 ±3.88	53.80 ±7.70
	EXP	48.14 ±12.72	50.67 ±7.84	47.39 ±11.39	48.51 ±8.64

* EXP > CON($F_{(9,1)}$ =3.66; p =0.08). No significance for all other SF12 scores. SF12: the 12-item short form health survey. PCS (SF12): physical component summary of SF12. MCS (SF12): mental component summary of SF12.

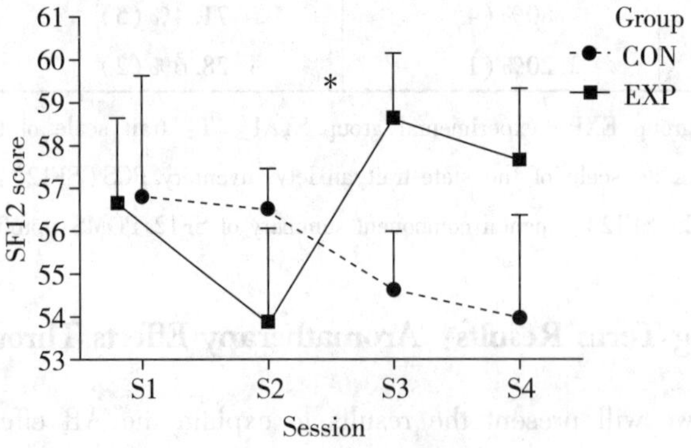

Figure 16 PCS(SF12) scores(Means and SD) in the 4 sessions(for both groups)

* EXP: significant increase. p =0.01(GLM).

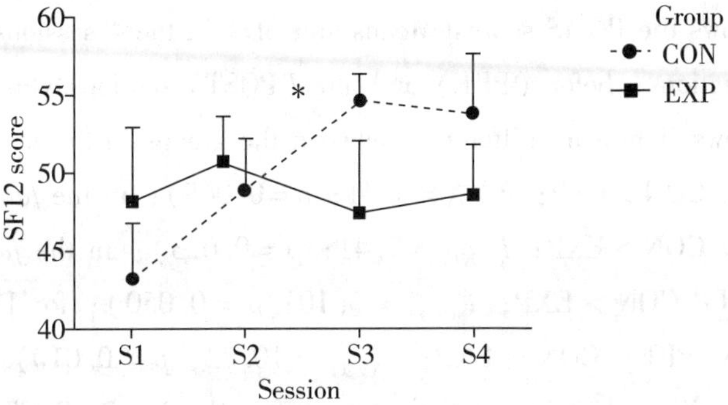

Figure 17 MCS(SF12) scores(Means and SD) in the 4 sessions(for both groups)

* CON: significant increase. $p = 0.03$ (GLM).

Table 7 shows the anxiety (STAI) and feeling scale (FACE) scores (Means and SD) in the 4 sessions of both groups and in both situations, before (PRE) and after (POST) sessions. One-way ANOVA for each session shows that the only significant difference between groups is before Session 4. In this session, EXP shows a bigger FACE_ PRE score than CON ($F_{(9,1)} = 8.18$; $p = 0.01$). There are no significant differences between groups into every session for all other PRE and POST scores, before and after sessions.

Table 7 STAI_ S and Feeling Scale scores(Means and SD) in the 4 sessions of Study 1(for both groups)

Quest	Group	Session 1	Session 2	Session 3	Session 4
STAI_ S_ PRE	CON	15. 50 ± 8. 73	15. 40 ± 5. 32	13. 00 ± 4. 30	23. 25 ± 4. 79
	EXP	16. 14 ± 10. 07	19. 71 ± 11. 32	9. 33 ± 6. 19	25. 28 ± 3. 04
STAI_ S_ POST	CON	14. 00 ± 10. 27	14. 60 ± 3. 64	9. 60 ± 7. 89	23. 00 ± 3. 91
	EXP	9. 43 ± 4. 35	13. 14 ± 6. 84	6. 83 ± 3. 54	24. 00 ± 2. 7
FACE_ PRE	CON	7. 33 ± 1. 03	7. 40 ± 0. 89	5. 60 ± 3. 21	6. 00 ± 0. 82
	EXP	7. 00 ± 1. 15	7. 00 ± 1. 29	7. 83 ± 1. 60	7. 43 ± 0. 79 *
FACE_ POST	CON	7. 50 ± 0. 83	6. 40 ± 2. 50	7. 60 ± 1. 14	7. 00 ± 0. 81
	EXP	7. 43 ± 0. 78	7. 43 ± 1. 27	8. 00 ± 1. 55	7. 71 ± 1. 4

* EXP > CON ($F_{(9,1)} = 8.18$; $p = 0.01$). STAI_ S: state scale of the state-trait anxiety inventory. PRE: previous period. POST: after inhalation period.

Table 8 shows the POMS scores(Means and SD) in the 4 sessions for both groups and for both situations, before(PRE) and after(POST) sessions. One-way ANOVA of each session shows significant difference between the groups in the *tension* score before Session 3(PRE: CON > EXP; $F_{(9,1)} = 5.41$; $p = 0.045$); in the *fatiguc* score before Session 3(PRE: CON > EXP; $F_{(9,1)} = 7.41$; $p = 0.023$); in the *fatigue* score after Session 3 (POST: CON > EXP; $F_{(9,1)} = 5.10$; $p = 0.050$); for POMS total score before Session 3 (PRE: CON > EXP; $F_{(9,1)} = 10.72$; $p = 0.010$). There is also a trend towards significance in the *fatigue* score after Session 2 (POST: CON > EXP; $F_{(10,1)} = 3.62$; $p = 0.086$); in the *fatigue* score before Session 4(PRE: CON > EXP; $F_{(9,1)} = 3.69$; $p = 0.087$); in the *vigor* score before Session 4(PRE: EXP > CON; $F_{(9,1)} = 3.71$; $p = 0.086$). There are no significant differences between all the other PRE and POST scores, before and after sessions.

Table 8 POMS scores(Means and SD) in the 4 sessions of Study 1(for both groups)

POMS scales	Group	Session 1	Session 2	Session 3	Session 4
Tension_ PRE	CON	2. 28 ±2. 16	2. 13 ±2. 66	2. 66 ±1. 13	4. 75 ±3. 84
	EXP	2. 24 ±2. 16	3. 52 ±2. 89	0. 50 ±0. 78 *	4. 52 ±2. 69
Tension_ POST	CON	0. 89 ±1. 42	1. 80 ±2. 26	1. 06 ±1. 68	1. 91 ±1. 16
	EXP	0. 33 ±0. 57	1. 86 ±1. 82	0. 27 ±0. 44	1. 95 ±2. 66
Hostility_ PRE	CON	0. 22 ±0. 40	0. 33 ±0. 47	0. 33 ±0. 58	0. 08 ±0. 17
	EXP	0. 29 ±0. 75	0. 62 ±1. 64	0. 22 ±0. 40	0. 43 ±0. 99
Hostility_ POST	CON	0. 11 ±0. 17			0. 33 ±0. 57
	EXP	0. 95 ±0. 25	0. 09 ±0. 25		0. 57 ±0. 99
Fatigue_ PRE	CON	2. 56 ±1. 66	3. 40 ±1. 09	2. 90 ±1. 80	3. 75 ±1. 32
	EXP	1. 81 ±1. 42	2. 33 ±2. 97	0. 72 ±0. 80	1. 19 ±2. 43 **
Fatigue_ POST	CON	1. 50 ±1. 24	3. 13 ±1. 99	1. 60 ±1. 47	3. 42 ±0. 83
	EXP	0. 62 ±0. 78	1. 24 ±1. 47 **	0. 22 ±0. 27 *	1. 14 ±2. 88
Depression_ PRE	CON	0. 90 ±0. 57	0. 33 ±0. 57	0. 60 ±0. 54	1. 58 ±1. 54
	EXP	1. 33 ±2. 82	1. 14 ±2. 04	1. 05 ±1. 25	0. 86 ±1. 99

续 表

POMS scales	Group	Session 1	Session 2	Session 3	Session 4
Depression_ POST	CON	0. 56 ±0. 75	0. 80 ±1. 26	0. 26 ±0. 43	0. 33 ±0. 38
	EXP	0. 38 ±0. 73	0. 67 ±1. 62	0. 27 ±0. 53	0. 67 ±1. 27
Vigor_ PRE	CON	6. 50 ±1. 05	5. 80 ±1. 87	5. 73 ±2. 06	4. 83 ±1. 89
	EXP	5. 95 ±1. 93	5. 38 ±2. 14	5. 83 ±1. 85	6. 5 ±1. 06**
Vigor_ POST	CON	5. 56 ±2. 56	5. 73 ±1. 80	6. 13 ±2. 98	4. 83 ±1. 89
	EXP	5. 42 ±1. 53	5. 47 ±2. 21	6. 00 ±2. 33	6. 52 ±1. 06
Total_ PRE	CON	4. 50 ±7. 76	4. 36 ±1. 01	4. 45 ±0. 52	5. 00 ±1. 31
	EXP	4. 32 ±1. 04	4. 72 ±1. 56	3. 36 ±0. 24*	4. 70 ±1. 47
Total_ POST	CON	3. 70 ±0. 54	4. 29 ±1. 28	3. 81 ±0. 54	4. 11 ±0. 64
	EXP	3. 37 ±0. 31	3. 86 ±0. 75	3. 35 ±0. 32	4. 09 ±1. 33

*$p<0.05$; **$p>0.05$ and $p<0.09$. PRE: previous period. POST: after inhalation period.

We did not put the data in Session 2, 3 and 4 of hostility_ POST is because there were too many artifacts in the HRV recordings.

We calculated the differences between the before and the after sessions for questionnaire scores to compare the evolution between groups through the 4 sessions. Table 9 shows the differences (Means and SD) between PRE and POST scores (PRE_ POST) in all questionnaires in the 4 sessions, for both groups. One-way ANOVA for each session shows a clear tendency to significance for STAI_ S difference score (DIF_ STAI_ S) in Session 2 (see Figure 18): EXP > CON ($F_{(10,1)}=4.37$; $p=0.063$). There is no significance for all other questionnaire scores.

Table 9 Differences (Means and SD) between PRE and POST scores (PRE_ POST) of all questionnaires in the 4 sessions (for both groups)

Questionnaires	Group	Session 1	Session 2	Session 3	Session 4
DIF_ STAI_ S	CON	1. 50 ±12. 01	0. 80 ±3. 11	3. 40 ±4. 09	0. 25 ±3. 40
	EXP	6. 71 ±6. 62	6. 57 ±5. 53	2. 50 ±3. 6	1. 28 ±1. 89

续 表

Questionnaires	Group	Session 1	Session 2	Session 3	Session 4
DIF_ FACE	CON	−0. 17 ±0. 40	1. 00 ±2. 83	−2. 00 ±3. 93	−1. 00 ±0. 81
	EXP	−0. 43 ±0. 79	−0. 43 ±0. 79	−0. 17 ±0. 40	−0. 29 ±1. 25
DIF_ tension	CON	1. 39 ±0. 88	0. 33 ±1. 17	1. 6 ±2. 07	2. 83 ±2. 98
	EXP	1. 90 ±1. 67	1. 6 ±1. 52	0. 22 ±0. 34	2. 57 ±1. 46
DIF_ hostility	CON	0. 11 ±0. 27	0. 33 ±0. 47	0. 33 ±0. 57	−0. 22 ±0. 69
	EXP	0. 19 ±0. 50	0. 52 ±1. 39	0. 22 ±0. 40	−0. 14 ±0. 69
DIF_ fatigue	CON	1. 06 ±1. 54	0. 26 ±1. 09	1. 33 ±1. 27	0. 33 ±1. 41
	EXP	1. 19 ±1. 17	1. 09 ±2. 02	0. 50 ±0. 58	0. 05 ±0. 59
DIF_ depression	CON	0. 38 ±0. 68	−0. 47 ±1. 28	0. 33 ±0. 47	1. 25 ±1. 52
	EXP	0. 95 ±2. 09	0. 47 ±0. 53	0. 78 ±1. 20	0. 19 ±0. 99
DIF_ vigor	CON	0. 94 ±1. 81	−0. 13 ±0. 76	−0. 40 ±2. 25	−0. 17 ±1. 03
	EXP	0. 52 ±0. 92	−0. 95 ±0. 68	−0. 17 ±1. 44	0. 38 ±1. 07
DIF_ total	CON	0. 78 ±0. 59	0. 07 ±0. 51	0. 64 ±0. 40	0. 40 ±0. 61
	EXP	0. 95 ±0. 85	0. 86 ±0. 91	0. 31 ±0. 30	0. 60 ±0. 44

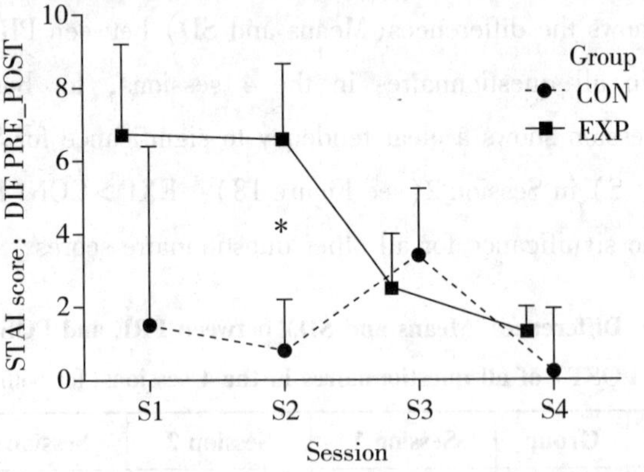

Figure 18　Differences between PRE and POST scores (PRE_ POST) for STAI _ S questionnaire in the 4 sessions(for both groups)

∗ EXP > CON; $p = 0.06$ (one-way ANOVA).

Table 10 shows the HRV parameters (Means and SD) in the 4 sessions for both groups and for both situations, before (PRE) and after (POST) sessions. One-way ANOVA for each session shows a trend towards significant difference between groups for HRmean after Session 3 (POST: CON > EXP; $F_{(10,1)} = 4.01$; $p = 0.073$), and for RRmean after Session 3 (POST: EXP > CON; $F_{(10,1)} = 3.66$; $p = 0.085$). There are no significant differences between groups in every session for all other HRV parameters, before and after the sessions.

Table 10 HRV parameters (Means and SD) in the 4 sessions (for both groups)

HRV	Group	Session 1	Session 2	Session 3	Session 4
HRmean_ PRE	CON	75.73 ± 9.19	79.26 ± 10.19	80.33 ± 8.57	
	EXP	69.53 ± 10.43	70.89 ± 11.75	73.13 ± 14.12	79.03 ± 9.34
HRmean_ POST	CON	75.77 ± 10.10	78.39 ± 13.65	80.29 ± 8.00	
	EXP	80.59 ± 39.67	67.25 ± 11.10	68.34 ± 11.41 **	70.61 ± 8.69
RRmean_ PRE	CON	828.72 ± 109.03	795.89 ± 111.23	780.80 ± 95.13	
	EXP	910.97 ± 136.76	901.67 ± 172.05	876.74 ± 172.46	791.46 ± 92.67
RRmean_ POST	CON	832.73 ± 131.16	814.13 ± 148.39	781.51 ± 83.73	
	EXP	866.68 ± 311.93	803.49 ± 344.17	934.00 ± 161.86 **	890.02 ± 112.19
SDRR_ PRE	CON	69.29 ± 16.81	62.76 ± 7.13	65.69 ± 20.69	
	EXP	72.74 ± 23.28	78.63 ± 33.07	62.33 ± 32.19	56.14 ± 22.37
SDRR_ POST	CON	69.42 ± 8.77	67.39 ± 15.08	74.05 ± 13.83	
	EXP	70.72 ± 19.67	80.36 ± 32.04	82.40 ± 29.07	88.89 ± 34.56
RMSSD_ PRE	CON	48.21 ± 15.47	36.94 ± 12.94	46.27 ± 22.80	
	EXP	51.04 ± 20.52	54.75 ± 35.13	49.11 ± 40.26	31.07 ± 13.80
RMSSD_ POST	CON	48.49 ± 14.85	43.59 ± 20.53	43.80 ± 11.95	
	EXP	53.39 ± 24.76	56.14 ± 33.43	62.87 ± 52.51	50.55 ± 12.58
LF/HF_ PRE	CON	1.52 ± 1.16	2.57 ± 1.34	2.90 ± 3.39	
	EXP	1.33 ± 1.19	1.70 ± 1.74	1.67 ± 1.38	1.86 ± 0.93

续 表

HRV	Group	Session 1	Session 2	Session 3	Session 4
LF/HF_ POST	CON	1.86 ±1.61	3.00 ±3.08	2.71 ±2.06	
	EXP	1.42 ±1.06	1.61 ±1.53	1.55 ±1.45	2.72 ±1.55
LFnu_ PRE	CON	53.70 ±19.18	69.37 ±9.16	59.34 ±25.66	
	EXP	48.83 ±21.93	52.01 ±23.73	52.24 ±25.81	62.03 ±11.44
LFnu_ POST	CON	55.83 ±19.18	63.33 ±20.88	64.77 ±19.67	
	EXP	49.95 ±24.54	50.05 ±25.77	50.59 ±24.27	68.57 ±14.32

** $p > 0.05$ and $p < 0.09$; [a] means for CON were not calculated because there were only 2 participants for this group in Session 4.

We calculated the difference between the results before and after the sessions for HRV parameters to compare the evolution between groups through the 4 sessions. Table 11 shows the differences (Means and SD) between PRE and POST parameters (PRE_ POST for HRmean; and POST_ PRE for all other parameters) in the 4 sessions for both groups. One-way ANOVA for each session shows a clear tendency to significance for the RRmean difference POST_ PRE (DIF_ RRmean) in Session 3: EXP > CON ($F_{(10,1)} = 3.94$; $p = 0.075$) (see Figure 19). There are no significant differences for all other HRV parameters.

Table 11 HRV parameters differences (Means and SD) between POST and PRE in the 4 sessions (for both groups: PRE_ POST for HRmean; and POST_ PRE for all other parameters)

HRV DIF	Group	Session 1	Session 2	Session 3	Session 4[a]
DIF_ HRmean	CON	-0.40 ±6.04	0.87 ±6.41	0.04 ±1.01	
	EXP	-11.05 ±40.70	3.64 ±1.81	4.79 ±6.25	8.42 ±7.19
DIF_ RRmean	CON	4.01 ±61.13	18.24 ±57.19	0.70 ±13.30	
	EXP	-44.28 ±230.95	-98.19 ±387.98	57.26 ±61.86 **	98.56 ±69.37
DIF_ SDRR	CON	0.13 ±10.57	4.63 ±12.84	8.36 ±20.87	
	EXP	-2.02 ±11.71	1.73 ±14.31	20.06 ±20.89	32.74 ±19.78

续 表

HRV DIF	Group	Session 1	Session 2	Session 3	Session 4
DIF_ RMSSD	CON	0. 28 ±17. 79	6. 66 ±10. 18	−2. 46 ±15. 19	
	EXP	2. 35 ±4. 43	1. 39 ±11. 26	13. 76 ±23. 50	19. 48 ±12. 43
DIF_ LF/HF	CON	0. 34 ±1. 01	0. 42 ±1. 82	−0. 20 ±3. 75	
	EXP	0. 09 ±0. 74	−0. 09 ±1. 64	−0. 12 ±1. 93	0. 86 ±1. 96
DIF_ LFnu	CON	2. 13 ±15. 4	−5. 70 ±14. 95	5. 43 ±19. 88	

** $p > 0.05$ and $p < 0.09$.

Means for CON were not calculated because there were only 2 participants for this group in Session 4.

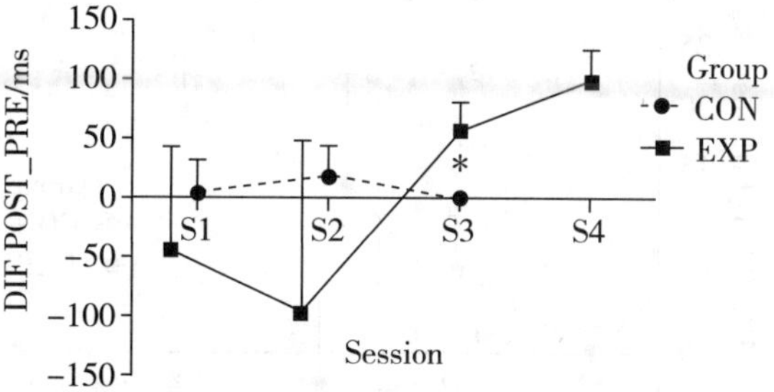

Figure 19 Differences between POST and PRE scores (POST _ PRE) for RRmean parameter in the 4 sessions(for both groups)

∗ EXP > CON; $p = 0.07$ (one-way).

Session 4 for CON was not included because there were only 2 participants.

Firstly, we analyzed the evolution of HRV parameters through the 4 sessions for EXP group with a GLM within-subjects' analysis. This analysis found a significant effect for the increasing DIF_ SDRR values(POST_ PRE) from Session 1 to Session 4(linear model; $F = 17.84$; $p = 0.006$) (see Figure 20). The same effect was observed on DIF_ RMSSD(POST_ PRE) from Session 1 to Session 4 (linear model; $F = 13.32$; $p = 0.011$) (see Figure 21). There were no significant differences in all the other HRV parameters.

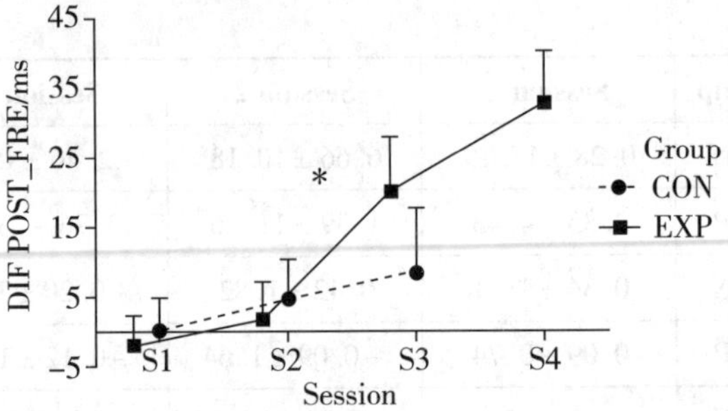

Figure 20　Differences between POST and PRE scores (POST_ PRE) for SDRR parameter in the 4 sessions(for both groups)

* EXP: significant increase. $p = 0.006$(GLM).

Session 4 for CON was not included because there were only 2 participants.

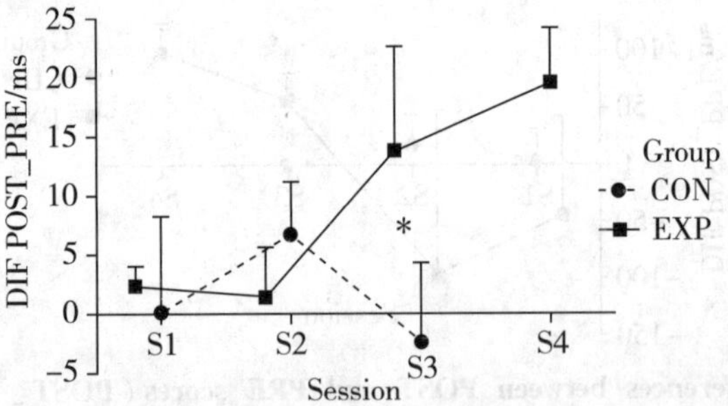

Figure 21　Differences between POST and PRE scores (POST_ PRE) for RMSSD parameter in the 4 sessions(for both groups)

* EXP: significant increase. $p = 0.006$(GLM).

Session 4 for CON was not included because there were only 2 participants.

Secondly, we analyzed the evolution of HRV parameters through the 3 sessions for CON with a GLM within-subjects' analysis(Session 4 for CON were not included because there were only 2 participants for this group in this session). There was no significance for any HRV parameters for CON.

5.5.3　Short Term Results: Aromatherapy Effects at 4 Periods

In this part we will present the results to explain the AR effects during the second session of the study. Seven participants completed the study for the experiment group and five for the control group. Nine participants did not complete the study because they could not attend 50% of the lab sessions. Table 5 shows the defining characteristics of the participants. There were no significant differences between the two groups in gender, age, physical activity level, anxiety trait (STAI), health perception (SF12) and academic performance. No significant differences between the two groups were found by HRV control variables like taking medicines, doing physical activity and drinking coffee. Thus, these results ensured that the participants of the two groups had equal characteristics.

Table 12 represents the comparison between the two groups about HRV parameters along the second session of the study, at baseline, at the 10 – 15 min, at the 20 – 25 min, at the 30 – 35 min and POST periods from the starting of smelling period. In this session, the essential oil for EXP was *Sweet basil* and the neutral oil for CON was *Sweet almond.*

Table 12　HRV parameters(M ± SD) for baseline(PRE), 10 –15 min(Dur 1), 20 –25 min(Dur 2) and 30 –35 min(Dur 3) in the second session of the study(for both groups)

HRV	Group	HR/bpm	RRmean/ms	SDRR/ms	RMSSD/ms	LF/ms^2
PRE	CON	76. 48 ±9. 86	795. 8 ±111. 23	62. 77 ±7. 13	37. 05 ±12. 98	1527. 98 ±524. 31
	EXP	68. 42 ±11. 45	901. 58 ±172. 99	73. 84 ±33. 22	50. 45 ±34. 47	1811. 56 ±2416. 53
Dur 1	CON	78. 34 ±10. 93	778. 61 ±114. 86	76. 58 ±18. 15	41. 21 ±15. 32	1336. 74 ±348. 21
	EXP	70. 09 ±9. 80	8871. 07 ±126. 61	89. 03 ±26. 83	48. 31 ±22. 16	1982. 38 ±1048. 29
Dur 2	CON	75. 92 ±13. 65	811. 58 ±149. 24	69. 33 ±18. 52	44. 24 ±21. 29	1437. 99 ±753. 99
	EXP	68. 20 ±9. 91	879. 49 ±142. 73	105. 59 ±29. 42	58. 66 ±34. 11 *	3768. 36 ±2810. 05
Dur 3	CON	75. 58 ±13. 05	814. 24 ±148. 31	67. 32 ±10. 99	43. 52 ±20. 77	1554. 86 ±745. 11
	EXP	67. 29 ±10. 99	914. 15 ±162. 58	84. 40 ±28. 91	51. 88 ±26. 79	1363. 71 ±990. 60
P(GLM)		NS	NS	0. 030	NS	0. 021

HRV	Group	HF/ms^2	VLF/ms^2	LF/HF	LFnu/ %	HFnu/ %
PRE	CON	734. 41 ±419. 15	1547. 08 ±628. 71	2. 6 ±1. 31	69. 66 ±9. 03	30. 35 ±9. 03
	EXP	1965. 89 ±3341. 73	2691. 46 ±3702. 61	1. 79 ±1. 94	52. 21 ±24. 27	47. 79 ±24. 27
Dur 1	CON	729. 21 ±307. 16	1693. 54 ±1033. 83	2. 35 ±1. 34	65. 62 ±14. 61	34. 38 ±14. 61
	EXP	841. 38 ±554. 01	3365. 05 ±2433. 62	2. 98 ±1. 76	68. 72 ±17. 26	31. 28 ±17. 26
Dur 2	CON	779. 33 ±487. 96	1857. 16 ±1197. 73	3. 17 ±2. 72	66. 15 ±20. 90	33. 85 ±20. 90
	EXP	1240. 76 ±1060. 55	7319. 75 ±5498. 00 *	6. 09 ±6. 34	73. 37 ±20. 68	26. 64 ±20. 68
Dur 3	CON	1178. 80 ±890. 32	1745. 32 ±1745. 37	2. 82 ±2. 99	62. 77 ±20. 07	37. 23 ±0. 06
	EXP	1582. 05 ±2039. 25	2561. 00 ±1977. 86	1. 58 ±1. 09	53. 61 ±22. 52	46. 39 ±22. 52
P(GLM)		NS	NS	NS	0. 015	0. 015

$*P < 0.05$；One-way.

The one-way ANOVA of each period shows a significant difference in Session 2 between groups for SDRR during 20 – 25 min period. In this period the EXP has a higher heart rate variability than CON (EXP > CON; $F_{(10,1)} = 5.84$; $p = 0.036$). EXP also shows higher VLF values than CON in Session 3 (EXP > CON; $F_{(10,1)} = 4.65$; $p = 0.05$). There are no significant differences between groups in any period for all the other HRV parameters.

An analysis of variance according to a general linear model shows differences between the two groups in terms of evolution throughout the 4 stages of the session (baseline, 10 – 15 min, 20 – 25 min and POS) for some HRV parameters. Thus, the EXP shows a significant peak at 20 – 25 min period for SDRR ($F_{(10,1)} = 6.35$; $p = 0.03$) (see Figure 22), LF ($F_{(10,1)} = 7.44$; $p = 0.021$) (see Figure 23) and LFnu ($F_{(10,1)} = 8.63$; $p = 0.015$) (see Figure 24) in comparison with CON; conversely proportional differences to LFnu are observed ($F_{(10,1)} = 8.63$; $p = 0.015$). There are no significant differences for all the other HRV parameters and periods.

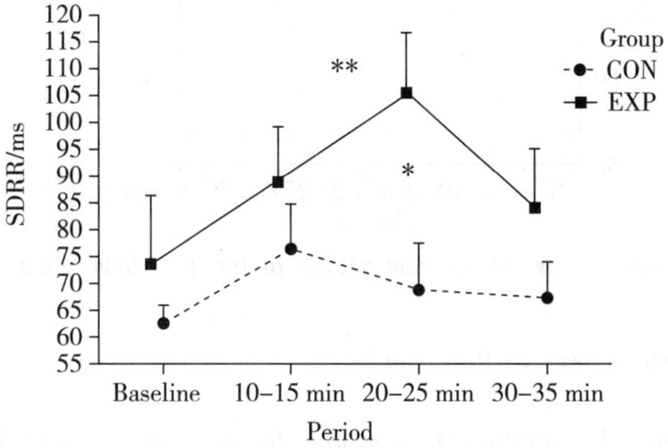

Figure 22 SDRR values (Means and SEM) in the 4 periods along Session 2 (for both groups)

* EXP > CON; $p = 0.036$ (one-way). ** EXP: significant peak, $p = 0.03$ (GLM). SEM: stand error of the mean (statistical parameter).

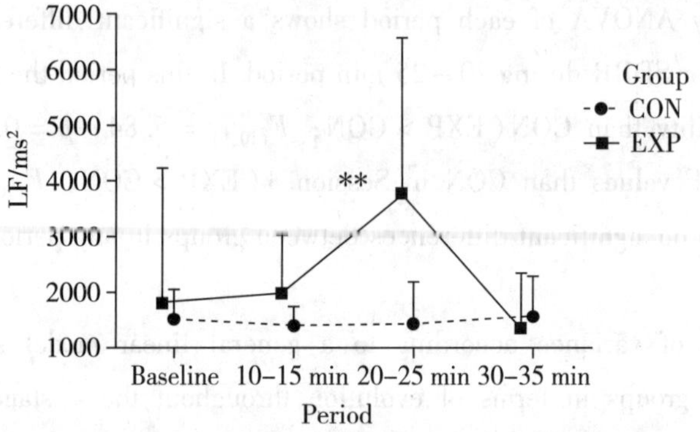

Figure 23 LF values(Means and SEM) in the 4 periods along Session 2(for both groups)

** EXP: significant peak. $p = 0.021$(GLM).

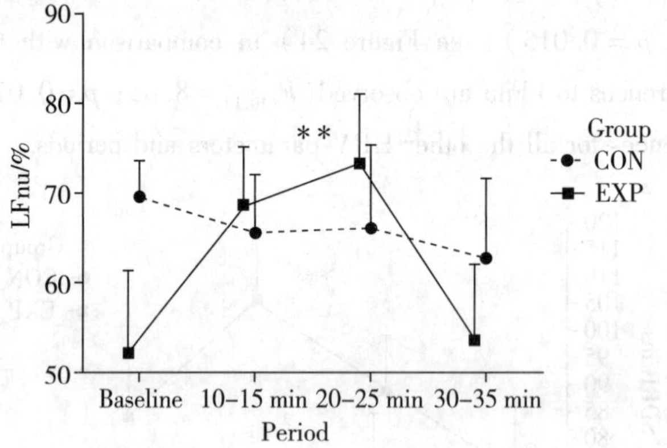

Figure 24 LFnu values(Means and SEM) in the 4 periods along Session 2(for both groups)

** EXP: significant peak. $p = 0.015$(GLM).

Table 13 shows the questionnaires scoring for both groups before(PRE) and after (POST) Session 2. We applied GLM analysis to compare the evolution from PRE to POST-session between both groups.

This analysis shows a significant difference between groups for STAI_ S scale, indicating that EXP shows a more pronounced decrease in POST than CON($F_{(10,1)} = 4.37$; $p = 0.05$)(see Figure 25). GLM also shows a tendency of significant difference between groups for *tension* scale(POMS) likewise($p = 0.98$)(see Figure 26). EXP also shows a more pronounced decrease in POST than CON in the same sense(but without statistical significant differences) for *depression* scale (POMS) (see Figure 27), and total POMS score (see Figure 28).

Table 13 Means and SD of the questionnaires scoring for both groups, before (PRE) and after (POST) Session 2

Variable	CON ($N=5$)	EXP ($N=7$)	p value
Anxiety (STAI_ S)			0. 050
Before	15. 40 ± 5. 31	19. 71 ± 11. 32	
After	14. 60 ± 3. 64	13. 14 ± 6. 84	
Total POMS			0. 120
Before	4. 36 ± 1. 01	4. 72 ± 1. 56	
After	4. 29 ± 1. 28	3. 86 ± 0. 75	
Tension (POMS)			0. 098
Before	2. 13 ± 2. 66	3. 52 ± 2. 89	
After	1. 80 ± 2. 25	1. 85 ± 1. 82	
Hostility (POMS)			NS
Before	0. 33 ± 0. 47	0. 61 ± 1. 63	
After	0. 00 ± 0. 00	0. 95 ± 0. 25	
Fatigue (POMS)			NS
Before	3. 40 ± 1. 09	2. 33 ± 2. 96	
After	3. 13 ± 1. 99	1. 23 ± 1. 47	
Depression (POMS)			0. 108
Before	0. 33 ± 0. 57	1. 14 ± 2. 04	
After	0. 80 ± 1. 26	0. 66 ± 1. 62	
Vigor (POMS)			NS
Before	5. 06 ± 1. 87	5. 38 ± 2. 13	
After	5. 73 ± 1. 80	5. 47 ± 2. 21	

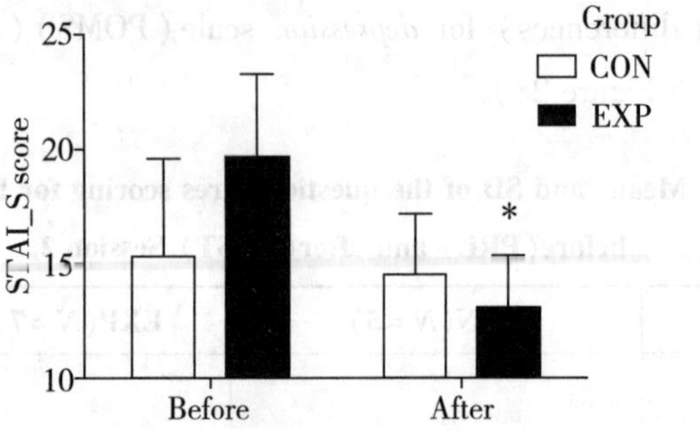

Figure 25　STAI_ S scores(Means and SEM) before and after Session 2(for both groups)

* EXP: significant decrease, $p = 0.05$ (GLM).

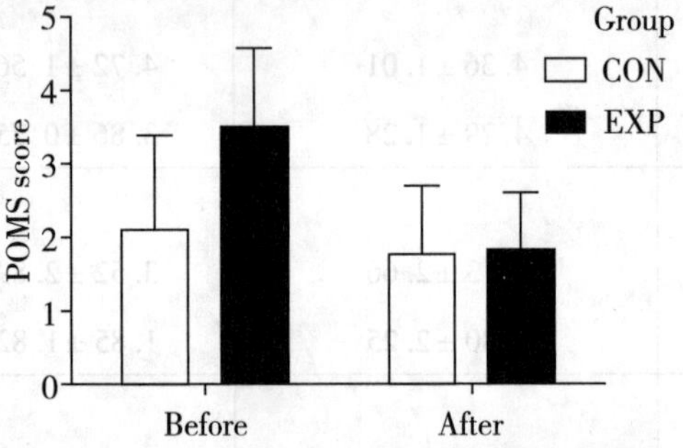

Figure 26　POMS *tension* scale scores(Means and SEM) before and after Session 2(for both groups)

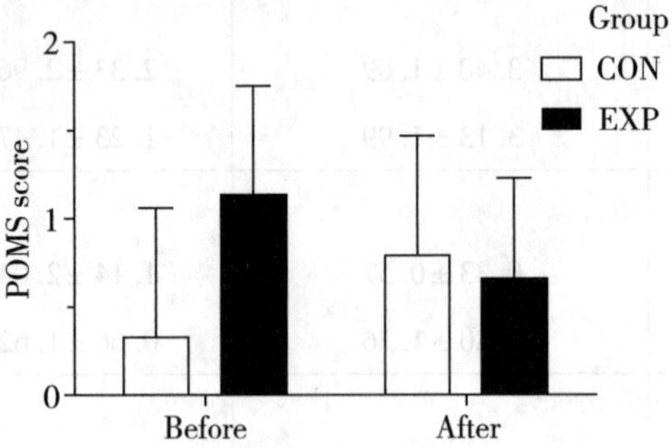

Figure 27　POMS *depression* scale scores(Means and SEM) before and after Session 2(for both groups)

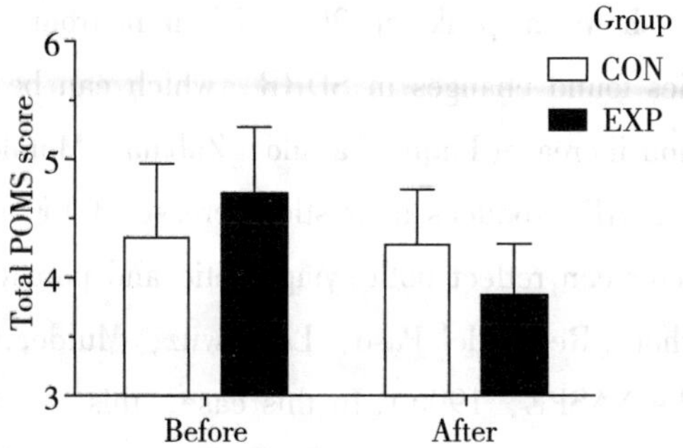

Figure 28 Total POMS scores(Means and SEM) before and after Session 2(for both groups)

5.6 Discussion

This study confirms the aromatherapy reduces university students' anxiety and increases their concentration in studying, not only in a short term period(45 min) but also in the long term(several weeks). Thus, the inhalation of *Sweet basil* oil through a short session or with an aromatic necklace every day during one month produces emotional and HRV changes on participants.

In this study, we have chosen a very common situation for university students all over the world: 1) A 45 min self-study session at their university school (in a lab situation); 2) One month in their students' life while they prepare a university exam at home. Overall, the results showed in the questionnaire scores indicated a reduction of anxiety and an increase of cardiac variability (tested through HRV analysis). These results can be explained by a balancing effect of AR on the sympathetic/parasympathetic system(ANS).

AR has short time effects because the inhalation of *Sweet basil* oil stimulates the sympathetic activity and increases the secretion of adrenaline. When comparing the experiment group and the control group, we can see that the experiment group showed a greater increase of the SDRR time domain parameter and LF and LFnu frequency domain parameters(see Figure 22, 23, 24). This incremental effect continued throughout the session. The SDRR effect can be interpreted by an increase of heart rate variability (Kudo, Shinohara, Kodama, 2014). In this case, it means that AR has a growing relaxing effect which shows a peak at 20 – 25 min from the beginning of the inhalation. Other studies found changes in SDRR, which can be explained by a stress reduction or a relaxation increase (Luque-Casado, Zabala, Morales, *et al.*, 2013).

At the same time, AR produces a drastic increase of LF and LFnu in the same period. The LF parameter can reflect both sympathetic and parasympathetic influences, according to other authors (Reyes del Paso, Langewitz, Mulder, *et al.*, 2013; Task Force of the ESC & the NASPE, 1996). In this case, this could be interpreted as an increase of the parasympathetic stimulation, which indicated that, compared to the CON, the EXP students could either experiment less negative emotions (like anxiety or stress) or experiment more positive emotions. In this case, high values in LF could also mean a positive sympathetic stimulation, interpreted as a rise of the arousal level (Luque-Casado, Zabala, Morales, *et al.*, 2013). Therefore, the short term action mechanism of AR can be explained by the balance of the ANS, which is caused by either an increment of the level of arousal (sympathetic activity), or by a reduction of the level of negative emotions (more heart rate variability and less anxiety). The given combination can facilitate the control of the attention level, a critical aspect for university students, whose studying require high levels of concentration. It is important to remark that this positive effect of AR reaches its peak at 20 – 25 min from the start of the *Sweet basil* oil inhalation and that this effect continues at least for 45 min (Haze Sakai, Gozu, 2002).

The questionnaires results confirm this action mechanism since the EXP shows a significant decrease of the anxiety level (STAI_ S) after Session 2 in comparison with the CON due to the effect of the *Sweet basil* oil inhalation (see Figure 25). This same effect can be observed through the decrease of other negative emotions such as *tension* scale, *depression* scale and total values for POMS (see Figure 26, 27 and 28).

The main result for the long time study is that *Sweet basil* oil inhalation seems to increase the heart rate variability and decrease the anxiety and the negative emotions through the 4 intervention weeks. In Figure 19, 20 and 21 we can observe that RRmean, SDRR and RMSSD show higher POST_ PRE increasing through the sessions for EXP. This increasing has not been observed for CON. This effect can be interpreted as an increase of cardiac variability due to the *Sweet basil* oil inhalation (Luque-Casado,

Zabala, Morales, *et al.*, 2013). The maximum HRV increase is produced in Session 3, when EXP have been inhaling *Sweet basil* oil for two weeks at home and have had three inhalation sessions in the lab. It could mean that AR has a growing relaxing effect which shows a maximum at 2 weeks from the beginning of the intervention. Other studies found changes in similar HRV parameters, which can be explained by a stress reduction or a relaxation increase (Chang, Shen, 2011).

The cognitive results analyzed by the questionnaires confirm this explanation. EXP showed significant lower values of negative emotions than CON in Session 2, 3 and 4, in POMS for total scoring or for scales like *tension* and *fatigue* (see Table 8). However, EXP showed higher values of *vigor*, the only positive POMS scale, accompanied by low values of *fatigue* for the last session (the exam day). The EXP also showed higher values than the CON of physical component summary (PCS) of SF12 for Session 3 and 4 (Figure 16). Thus, it seems that *Sweet basil* oil improves the perception of better wellness about physical aspect, especially at long term after 2 weeks. It is especially important in Session 4 because it is the exam day for all the participants and this wellness questionnaire was used just before starting the exam. After 3 – 4 weeks of *Sweet basil* oil inhalation, the students felt more active, healthier and less tired. It could be interpreted as an improving effect on the arousal. This state together with a better control over the negative emotion might be appropriate to achieve enough concentration to copy with exams. In fact, the students felt better before the exam when they inhaled *Sweet basil* oil the previous weeks (see the results for the Feeling Scale in Session 4, Table 7).

After this results we concluded that the use of aromatherapy can be useful to reduce academic anxiety, to improve students' concentration, and it might not only improve academic performance in a relatively short time (one session) but also at long time (one month). Other investigations support our findings indicating that short term aroma inhalation modulates HRV with the predominance of sympathetic nervous system activity while inducing soothing effects and reducing anxiety (Saeki, 2000). Demonstrated significant changes in HRV parameters related with sympathovagal balance and associated with relaxation at 5 min after the completion of a foot bath with lavender oil. We found that the HRV parameters changed around 20 – 25 min after starting the inhalation. In this sense, Kuroda, *et al.* (2005) found that HF power increased more significantly at 21 min than after a 6 min olfactory stimulation of linalool. In the same line, we found major changes at 20 – 25 min after starting the inhalation. In one of their studies, Satou, Chikama M, Chikama Y, *et al.* (2013) found that an aromatherapy massage could be effective on elderly patients under long term hospitalization. Meanwhile, Matsumoto and his colleagues (2013) found that lavender aromatherapy alleviates premenstrual emotional symptoms with a 3-month intervention. Finally, Igarashi and his colleagues (2014) found that the stimulation with rose and orange oil on the prefrontal cortex activity produces agitation.

The current findings proving that protective aroma effects reduce negative emotions add to increasing evidence supporting that some aromas may protect cognitive functions. The presence of essential oils and their composition determine the specific effects of plants on emotions. For example, for *Sweet basil* essential oil, this effect can be explained by the combined action of *Sweet basil* main components. Some of these essential oil components have sedative effects related to Yin (see Figure 4), such as esters, sesquiterpene hydrocarbons, linalyl acetate and linalool. These components can induce changes on the parasympathetic activity. Some of the essential oil components have activation effects related to Yang, such as phenol, aldehyde, oxides. These components can induce changes on the sympathetic activity. Some of the essential oil components have activation effects related to Yang and Yin, they can have both an activation and a sedative effect. The use of high components concentration could have activation effects. Unlike, the use of low components concentration could have sedative effects. In Figure 14 we can observe the *Sweet basil* main components: linalool (40% – 55%), methyl chavicol (7%) and phenol 6%. Methyl chavicol is a kind of phenylpropanoid with specific chemical qualities related to Yang, but it has a balance effect on the autonomic nervous system. Haze, *et al.* (2002) found that methyl chavicol induced stimulation of sympathetic activity. In the same sense, Schnaubelt (1998) confirmed that the phenylpropane ethers, especially estragole (methyl chavicol) stabilize an overactive sympathetic nervous system (sympatholytic effect) and restore a healthy balance between the sympathetic and parasympathetic nervous systems. Linalool is another component in aroma that could have some activation effects by stimulating the sympathetic activity. Linalool is a natural enantiomer monoterpene commonly found as the major volatile component of essential oils in several aromatic plant species, which is known to exhibit several biological activities such as CNS depressant, antinociceptive, anxiolytic and anticonvulsant(Peana, *et al.*, 2002; Peana, *et al.*, 2006; Kamatou, *et al.*, 2008). Other authors indicated the use of *Sweet basil* as a sedative in Spain (Vázquez, *et al.*, 1997) and as a sedative and anticonvulsant in Mexico(Tortoriello, Romero, 1992). Together with vitamin C, carotene, calcium and phosphorus, it also ensures skin health and tonicity of the nervous system, consolidating the memory processes. Eugenol is another kind of chemical component in *Sweet basil* oil. It is a phenylpropene, an allyl chain-substituted guaiacol. Eugenol is a member of the phenylpropanoids classes of chemical components. It could also be found as a chemical component in clove oil, nutmeg, cinnamon, basil and bay leaf. Eugenol also has been used in traditional medical systems to relieve symptoms and cure a variety of diseases (Peana, *et al.*, 2002). It also has an adaptive role, with antistress effect, it helps nervous and emotional processes, and it has an immunostimulant effect. Robin, *et al.* (1999) have shown that basic emotions evoked by eugenol odor differ according to the dental experience. One possible explanation of the stimulating effect of the components of *Sweet basil* could be that the oil(absorbed via the olfactory system) stimulates the locus coeruleus in the brain into releasing noradrenalin, a neurotransmitter that creates a stimulating/activating effect. The locus coeruleus is also involved in arousal and activation processes. Another possible explanation of its effect could be that *Sweet basil* exerts its effects by an interaction with central structure (e. g. hypothalamic, limbic, thalamic) which controls the level of autonomic and/or behavioral arousal. Overall, our study agrees with the importance of *Sweet basil* as a way to reduce anxiety, raise the level of positive emotion and improve quality of study in university students.

The chemical components of *Sweet basil* oil might help the participants' body to obtain a balanced status. Thus, essential oils can have certain "vitality" that helps our body to achieve a healthy state. According to TCM, essential oils can work through a truly holistic therapy, taking into account the mind, the body and the spirit of the person. Essential oils can connect with our bodies and help it to find the best way to solve our bodies need. In this case, the final effect can be an improvement of the mental and emotional condition by a combination of reducing the anxiety level before and during an exam and increasing the arousal level of the participants in terms of attentiveness and alertness.

5.7 Conclusion

With the aid of HRV analysis, our study confirms that *Sweet basil* inhalation can reduce anxiety level and increase study concentration of university students at short time (one-hour session) and long time (one month). The EXP reduced academic anxiety level and incremented cardiac variability compared to the CON. These results could be explained by an autonomic balance on the sympathetic/parasympathetic system through a combined action of the *Sweet basil* components: linalool (40% – 55%), methyl chavicol (7%) and phenol (6%). Some of these components have sedative effects. tif (parasympathetic activity), which belong to Yin in TCM, and others can have activation effects (sympathetic activity), which pertain to Yang in TCM.

6 Study for Determining Whether Aroma Improves Work Performance and Reduces Workplace Stress

6. 1 Objective

The purpose of this chapter is to conduct a pilot study for determining the procedures and characteristics of aroma methods, whether aroma improves work performance and reduces workplace stress. This information will be useful to conduct the definitive Study 2.

6. 2 Sample

The participants were 5 university professors who used to sit in front of computers several hours per day (3 males and 2 females; aged from 30 to 53). All participants consented to collaborate voluntarily and provided informed consent before participating in the pilot study. They met the following inclusion criteria: 1) no clinical diagnosis of autonomic dysfunction; 2) no clinical diagnosis of respiratory, cardiovascular, endocrine or systemic disorder; 3) no problems with olfactory function; 4) none of the participants had been clinically diagnosed with diabetes mellitus, hypertension, hyperlipidemia, asthma, cardiovascular disorders, or any other endocrine or systemic disorders that could affect the autonomic nervous system. All five participants completed a total of 6 sessions in a lab or workplace situation.

6. 3 Instruments

For this pilot study we used the FitLab Team system (see Chapter 3 Section 2) to analyze HRV, and the questionnaire STAI_ S, POMS, SF_ 12v2 and the Feeling Scale (see Chapter 3 Section 1).

6. 4 Specific Procedure for Pilot Study 2

We did not inform participants about which fragrance or oil we would use for the study.

We conducted this pilot study through 6 sessions in different weeks and conditions (see Table 14).

Table 14 Characteristics for the 6 sessions conducted in the Pilot Study 2 with university staff

Session	Participants	Time	Place	Status	Aroma	Use way
Session 1	5	60min	Lab	Working	CAB	Inhaling
Session 2	5	60min	Office	Working	CAB	Inhaling
Session 3	5	60min	Lab	Working	CL	Inhaling
Session 4	5	60min	Office	Working	CL	Inhaling
Session 5	5	60min	Office	Working	CAB	Inhaling
Session 6	5	60min	Office	Working	CL	Inhaling

CAB: *Citrus aurantium bigarade* (*Petitgrain*). CL: *Canarium luzonicum* (*Elemi*).

The participants went to the lab in 2 group sessions distributed in different weeks. Those sessions were performed in the morning between 9:00 and 11:00 in a lab quiet environment. The ambient temperature was controlled between 22℃ and 25℃. The other 4 sessions were performed at the participants' individual work site and they were working in a sitting position in front computers between 9:00 and 11:00.

In general, the intervention consisted in a 45 min aroma inhalation of a specific kind of oil *Elemi* (CL) and *Petitgrain* (CAB). All participants performed a total of 6 sessions in 6 weeks. All participants were asked not to consume any food of beverages containing alcohol or caffeine after the evening of the day preceding the study sessions. They were also asked not to do vigorous physical activity during 24 hours before testing. Participants arrived at lab or their office and they were asked to rest in a sitting position in front of a table. In general, they followed these steps:

1) Participants were required to fill out the PRE questionnaires (STAI_ S, POMS, SF_ 12v2) and the Feeling Scale.

2) Participants were asked to wear the cardiac chest band (connected via bluetooth to an iPad with FitLab software) and sit at rest in front of the table.

3) HRV_ PRE (before aroma inhale) was recorded for 5 minutes with the participants at this rest situation: sitting, opening eyes, putting hands on their knees,

doing no activity, breathing naturally and speaking nothing.

4) Participants were asked to do a usual work task but in a quiet situation and without speaking to each other. Participants kept this work situation during all the sessions. Meanwhile, they were inhaling the oil aroma and the HRV was being recorded during the session. The HRV was recorded in a three 5 min periods: During 1, at 10 – 15 min from inhalation starting; During 2, at 20 – 25 min; and During 3, at 30 – 35 min.

5) Participants were required to perform a 5 min HRV posttest (sitting, opening eyes, putting hands on their knees, doing no activity, breathing naturally and speaking nothing).

6) Participants were asked to fill out the POST questionnaires (STAI_ S, POMS and the Feeling Scale).

6.5 Results

In this part we presented only the most relevant results of this pilot study for obtaining the key information to design the definitive Study 2 (Chapter 7). Five participants completed the study. The initial participants were university professors of different ages and both sexes and they had to inhale different aroma characteristics in a heterogenic. All participants showed a sufficient compliance with the HRV control variables like no taking medicines, doing low level of physical activity and no drinking coffee before HRV analysis.

In order to check the aromatherapy efficacy to improve work performance and reduce workplace stress, we analyzed the effects of inhaling *Elemi* (CL) and *Petitgrain* (AB) on HRV through Session 3, 4, 6 and 1, 2, 5 respectively. We performed HRV analysis before, during and after the 6 sessions of the pilot study.

Table 15 shows the HRV parameters at baseline (PRE), 10 – 15 min (During 1), 20 – 25 min (During 2), 30 – 35 min (During 3) and after the inhalation period (POST). The values are means (and SD) for the 5 participants and for the 3 sessions corresponding to each oil (*Elemi* and *Petitgrain*).

A visual inspection of the results shows some differences between both oils in HRV parameters at different intra-session periods.

Table 15 HRV parameters(Means and SD) for the 5 participants in the 5 session periods

Aroma	Time	RRmean/ms	SDRR/ms	RMSSD/ms	LF/HF	LFnu/%	HFnu/%
CAB	PRE	965.60±169.65	80.26±40.89	62.87±49.01	2.99±2.17	67.44±21.45	32.5±21.45
	Dur 1	956.98±173.145	46.90±31.02	42.03±34.40	2.88±1.64	70.67±11.57	29.39±11.48
	Dur 2	945.98±166.03	88.17±54.85	55.62±44.03	3.56±2.68	66.91±24.98	33.09±24.98
	Dur 3	928.76±174.47	90.44±45.78	57.55±41.98	5.22±3.58	73.68±22.31	26.31±22.31
	POST	915.64±136.01	98.44±53.20	52.55±36.63	6.08±4.83	76.40±18.48	23.60±18.48
CL	PRE	853.83152.56	81.91±49.19	58.40±21.16	2.90±3.12	63.33±18.38	36.76±18.39
	Dur 1	876.59±156.87	66.59±38.72	46.92±31.92	4.00±3.95	61.50±17.86	38.49±17.86
	Dur 2	872.93±152.74	57.72±29.03	31.53±15.31	2.6±2.26	65.52±14.53	34.37±14.53
	Dur 3	887.94±169.57	67.57±31.52	53.59±35.23	2.08±1.73	55.72±24.78	44.27±24.77
	POST	897.40±191.98	82.88±18.50	68.07±30.87	1.71±1.37	57.52±15.09	42.48±15.09

PRE: before inhalation. Dur 1: at 10 – 15min after the inhalation started. Dur 2: at 20 – 25min. Dur 3: at 30 – 35min. POST: after inhalation. CL: *Elemi* inhalation (Session 3, 4 and 6); CAB: *Petitgrain*(Session 1, 2 and 5). Dur: during.

LF/HF increases at 20 – 25 min, 30 – 35 min and POST for *Petitgrain*, meanwhile it decreases in all these periods for *Elemi*(see Figure 29). Thus, the aroma inhalation seems to have an opposite effect over sympathetic/parasympathetic balance (LF/HF) from 10 – 15 min to the end of the inhalation.

SDRR decreases more at 10 – 15 min when inhaling *Petitgrain* than inhaling *Elemi*, and increases more at 20 – 25 min than inhaling *Elemi* (see Figure 30). *Petitgrain* maintains higher SDRR values than *Elemi* at 30 – 35 min and POST indicating more heart variability for the first one.

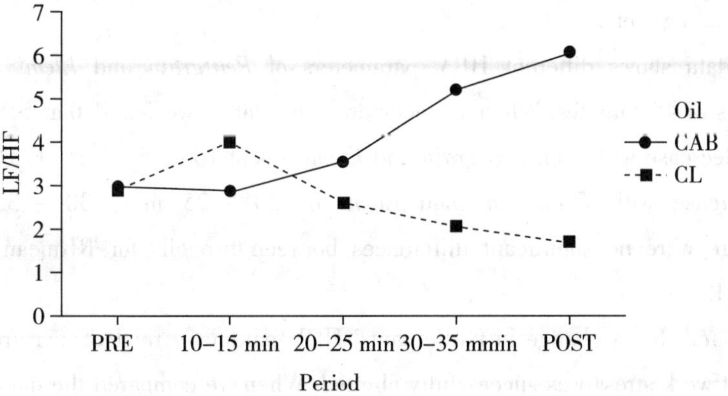

Figure 29 LF/HF mean for the 5 participants in the 5 session periods(PRE-inhalation; at 10 – 15min from inhalation starting; at 20 – 25min; at 30 – 35min; and POST, after inhalation)[for *Elemi* inhalation(CL; Session 3, 4 and 6) and *Petitgrain* (CAB; Session 1, 2 and 5) inhalation]

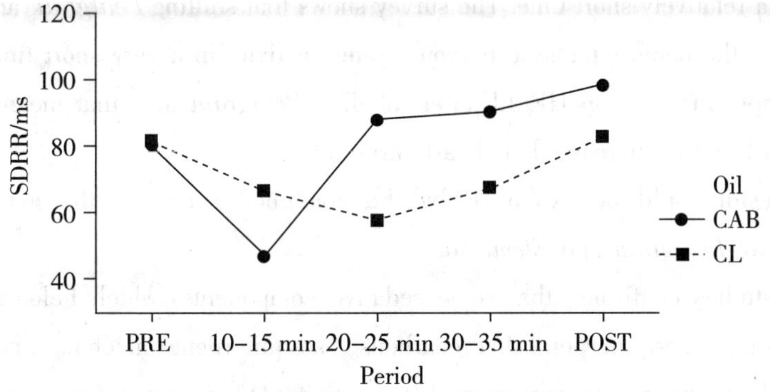

Figure 30 SDRR mean for the 5 participants in the 5 session periods(PRE-inhalation; at 10 – 15min from inhalation starting; at 20 – 25min; at 30 – 35min and POST, after inhalation)[for *Elemi* inhalation(CL; Session 3, 4 and 6) and *Petitgrain*(CAB; Session 1, 2 and 5) inhalation]

6.6 Discussion

The pilot study evaluated the effects that *Petitgrain* and *Elemi* oil have on reducing the level of stress in the workplace and improving work performance. To evaluate these two parameters, we used HRV analysis. We have evaluated these effects on very common situations of administrative university workers: working with computers, writing, reading, etc.

This data shows different HRV parameters of *Petitgrain* and *Elemi* after aroma stimulations of 45 minutes. When we compared the data, we found that SDRR showed the same decrease with both *Petitgrain* and *Elemi* oils at 10 – 15 min; LF/HF showed a higher increase with *Petitgrain* than *Elemi* at 20 – 25 min, 30 – 35 min and POST. There were no significant differences between two oils for RRmean, RMSSD, HFnu and LFnu.

We found that a change in participants' HRV-parameter related measures following a battery of work stress was successfully elicited. When we compared the data before and after inhaling the aroma, we found that the HRV parameters had changed. We also found that after inhaling the aroma of *Petitgrain* and *Elemi* oil for a period of 45 minutes, the stress in the workplace could be reduced and work performance could improve in a relatively short time. The survey shows that sniffing *Petitgrain* and *Elemi* oil can stimulate the parasympathetic nervous system activity in a very short time. The data shows a deeper increase on HF/LF after inhaling *Petitgrain* oil, that means *Petitgrain* oil could be trend to increase their heart variability.

This result could be explained by the combined action of the main chemical composition of *Petitgrain* and *Elemi* oil.

Some studies confirmed that some sedative components (which belongs to Yin), such as esters, sesquiterpene hydrocarbons, sesquiterpene alcohols and lactones, etc. may induce changes in parasympathetic activity. Other components can have some activation effects by stimulating the sympathetic activity. It could be explained to Yang. (Haze, Sakai, Gozu, 2002)

The predominant constituents of *Petitgrain* are linalyl acetate, linalool and myrcene (see Figure 31). Some of these components, such as linalyl acetate and linalool, have a sedative effect, which could induce changes on the parasympathetic activity (Kuroda, Inoue, Ito, *et al.*, 2005). Myrcene is another component in aroma plants that could have some activation effects by stimulating the sympathetic activity. Myrcene, a kind of monoterpene (1.3% – 2.12%), could possibly be related to the release of norepinephrine, a neurotransmitter linked to the sympathetic activity stimulation (Franchomme, Jollois, Penoel, 2001). The predominant constituents of *Elemi* are phellandrenes, elemenes, elemol (Franchomme, Jollois, Penoel, 2001) (see Figure 31).

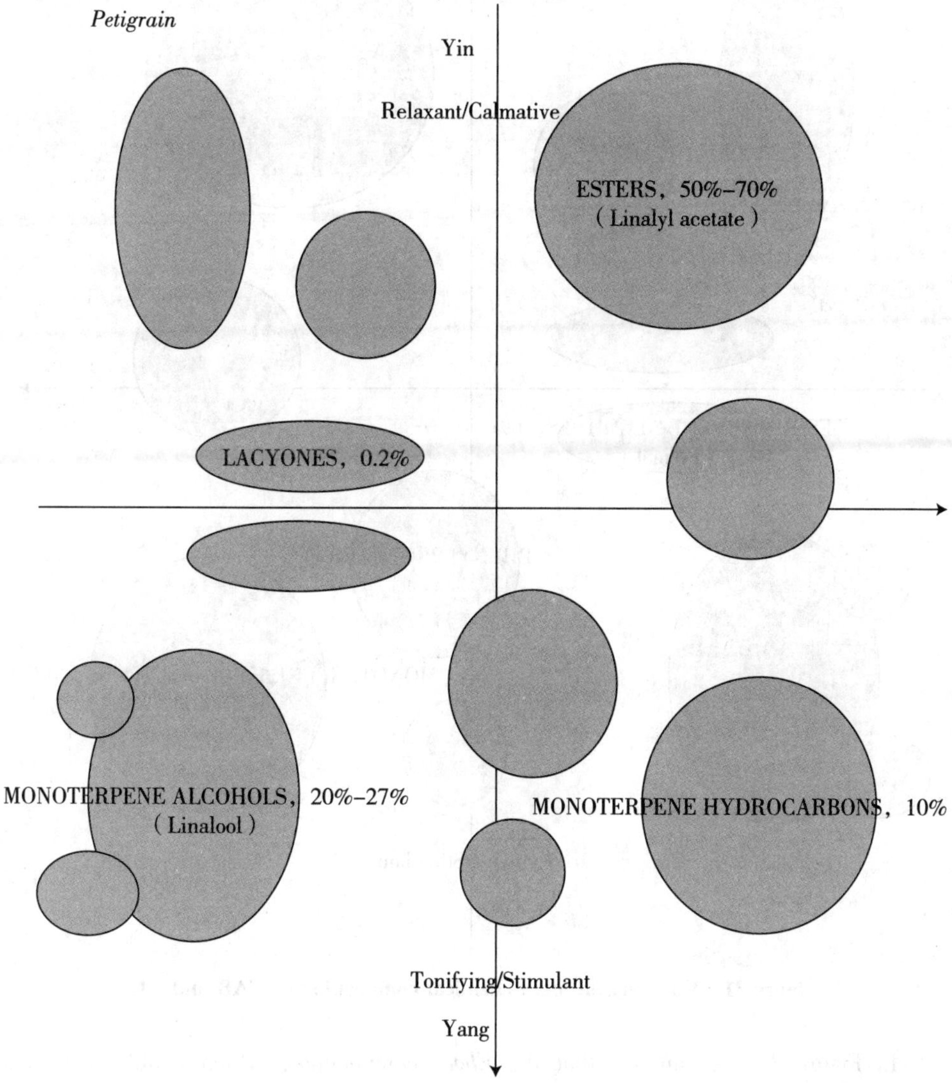

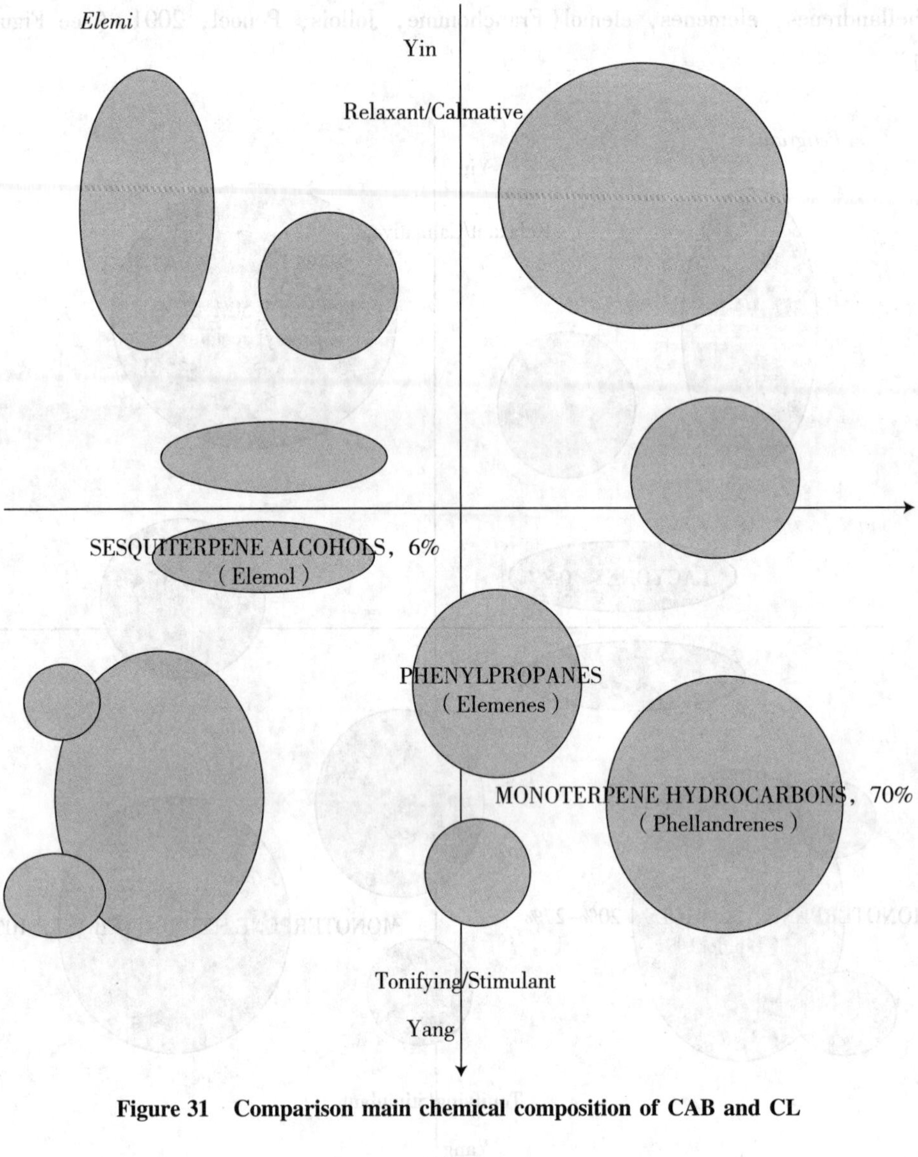

Figure 31　Comparison main chemical composition of CAB and CL

In Figure 31 we can see that the *Elemi* components, which could have some activation effects by stimulating the sympathetic activity, belong to Yang; while the *Petitgrain* main components can be found both in Yin and Yang(Franchomme, Jollois, Penoel, 2001).

The olfactory neuroanatomy is intertwined via extensive reciprocal axonal connections, frontal cortex and other parts of the limbic system. The odor molecules of essential oils are transmitted to the brain by olfactory sensory neurons in the nasal cavity. Thus, they stimulate smell-memory work and influence memory, thoughts, and emotions(Krusemark, Novak, Gitelman, *et al.*, 2013).

The limited of this study is the living habits of participants affected the rule of experimental requirements, such as drinking coffee in the morning. Despite repeated reminders, some participants did not perform well.

We also found that all the oils are useful for participants to improve a negative emotion. We may conduct another study to research on other essential oils in the future.

6.7 Conclusion

We have analyzed *Petitgrain* and *Elemi* HRV parameters, we found that the HF/LF value of *Petitgrain* oil was higher than that of *Elemi* oil. Recently, some researchers claimed that *Petitgrain* has sedative and anxiolytic like effects, such as the work of Lehrner, Christine Eckersberger, Walla, *et al.*, They found that *Petitgrain* reduced the anxiety level of patients, specifically women, when this kind of oil was scattered in the lobby of a dental office. Another study showed that *Petitgrain* oil(administered orally and derived from the petals and stamens) reduced the preoperative anxiety of patients scheduled for elective minor surgery.

In Figure 31, we can see how *Elemi* components are closer to Yang and it could have some activation effects by stimulating the sympathetic activity; while *Petitgrain* main components belong both to Yin and Yang. That means the chemical components of *Petitgrain* provide more balance than that of *Elemi* (see the structure-effect diagram of essential oils in Figure 31).

The study was focused on determining whether *Petitgrain* and *Elemi* can be used to improve work performance and reduce workplace stress. The results of this study showed that *Petitgrain* works better to balance the sympathetic/parasympathetic system and improve negative emotion.

7 Aroma Improves Work Performance and Reduces Workplace Stress

7.1 Objective

The purpose of this chapter is to analyze the efficacy of aromatherapy to improve work performance and reduce workplace stress. Specifically, we will check the effects of smelling *Patitgrain* on a simulated computer work session to improve the performance time when typing on the keyboard. At the same time, we will analyze the possible effects over HRV and mood/anxiety state questionnaires to explain the results in terms of sympathetic/parasympathetic balance, stress reduction and changes of arousal or attention level.

7.2 Sample

42 administrative university workers composed of the initial sample (age: 42.21 years, SD = 7.12; gender: 10 males and 32 females). All participants met the following inclusion criteria: 1) age between 26 and 55 years; 2) no clinical diagnosis of autonomic dysfunction; 3) no clinical diagnosis of respiratory, cardiovascular, endocrine or systemic disorder; 4) no problems with olfactory function. All participants consented to collaborate voluntarily and provided informed consent before participating in the study. The ethics committee of the university approved the study in advance.

A randomized controlled trial was used. The participants were recruited from a university administrative staff through an institutional email advertisement. All of them were used to working sitting and typing in front of computers for most of the working days. The participants were randomly assigned to the experiment group (EXP) and the control group (CON), and they were invited on different days to participate in specific sessions for each group. They were not aware of which group they were assigned. Explanations were provided regarding the nature and purpose of the study: to investigate coping effects of plant fragrance on workplace stress. All participants were asked not to consume any food or beverage containing alcohol or caffeine after the evening of the day preceding the experiment. They were also asked not to do vigorous physical activities during 24 hours before testing.

7.3 Instruments

For this study we used the FitLab Team system (see Chapter 3 Section 2) to analyze HRV and the questionnaire STAI_ S, POMS and the Feeling Scale (see Chapter 3 Section 1). The participants inhaled the essential oils through four diffusers that allowed a proper smelling throughout the room. We used two kinds of oils, one for each group: 1) EXP inhaled *Petitgrain* (*Citrus aurantium bigarade*. Abbreviation: CAB. 100% pure CAB was used and diluted to 2%. The predominant constituents were linalyl acetate (45% - 55%), linalool (20% - 27%) and myrcene (1.3% - 12.12%). 2) CON inhaled *Sweet almond* oil (*Prunus amygdalus* var. *dulcis*. Abbreviation: PAD. American, Production batch: YA637, Neroly Company Limited, Hong Kong). The predominant constituents were palmitoleic acid (60% - 68%), linoleic acid (17% - 30%) and palmitic acid (6% - 8%). PAD is a vegetable oil and has a neutral effect for smelling.

7.4 Procedure

We randomly distributed the participants into 6 sessions (7 subjects each) in different days, 3 for EXP and 3 for CON. All sessions were performed in a university computer classroom between 10: 00 and 11: 30 and each participant came only once. When the participants arrived at the computer classroom, they were asked to wear the cardiac chest band (bluetooth connected) and to rest in a sitting position in front of a computer, like in their workplace. Firstly, participants were required to fill out the questionnaire STAI_ S, POMS and the Feeling Scale. Secondly, HRV_ PRE was tested for 5 minutes with the participants at rest (sitting, opening eyes, placing their hands on their knees, doing no activity, breathing naturally and speaking nothing). Third, at the end of HRV_ PRE test, the oil diffusers were launched and worked throughout the session with CAB for EXP sessions and PAD for CON sessions (Figure 32, Step A). At the same time, a researcher explained for about 15 min how to complete a neutral computer task in a specific website (see Figure 32).

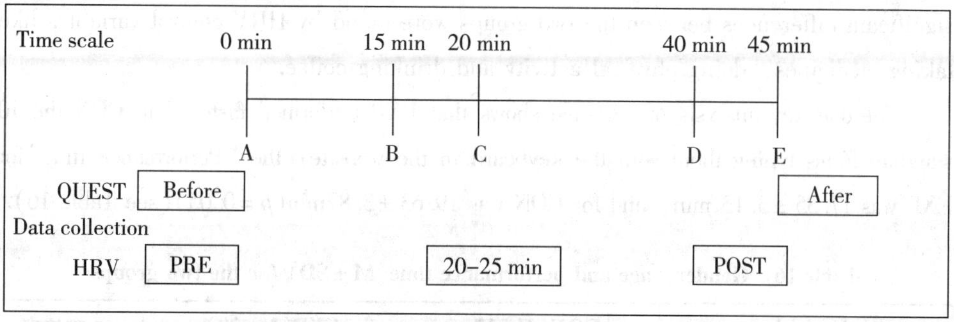

Figure 32 Experimental procedures and data collection

Before: STAI _ S and POMS questionnaires. PRE: 5 min HRV _ PRE Test. A: inhalation beginning. B: computer task beginning. C: 5 min HRV (20 – 25 min) test. D: computer task finishing (individual"Performance time"). POST: 5 min HRV post test(step D to E). After: STAI_ S and POMS.

This task was the same for all participants and consisted on completing 10 standard forms. All participants began individually to complete this task typing on their keyboard until they finished it(Step B to Step D in Figure 32). The single times(Step B to Step D) were different for all participants and were recorded in the website as"Performance time". A period of 5 min-HRV(Step C) was recorded at 20 – 25 min from the beginning of the inhalation period(Step A). Forty minutes after the inhalation beginning(Step A), all participants had finished their website task and their HRV was recorded during a period of 5 min (POST; Step D to E) in the same conditions as the HRV _ PRE. Finally, participants were asked to fill out the POST questionnaires(STAI_ S, POMS and the Feeling Scale).

7.5 Results

Among the 42 initial participants, 5 did not complete the study because they showed too many artefacts in the HRV recordings. For the EXP, 20 out of 21 participants completed the study, and for CON the number of participants was 17 out of 21. There were no statistically significant differences between EXP and CON in age (EXP: 43.0 ±6.4 years old. CON: 43.2 ±6.8 years old) or gender(EXP: 20% of male and 80% of female. CON: 31.6% of male and 68.4% of female), and no significant differences between the two groups were found by HRV control variables like taking medicines, doing physical activity and drinking coffee.

The one-way analysis of variance shows that EXP performed faster than CON the 10 standard forms typing them with the keyboard in the website: the "Performance time" for EXP was 17.35 ±3.13 min, and for CON was 19.63 ±3.87min ($p = 0.05$) (see Table 16).

Table 16 Gender, age and performance time (M ± SD) for the two groups

Variable	CON (*N* = 17)	EXP (*N* = 20)	*p* value
Age (years)	43.21 ±6.80	43.00 ±6.44	NS
Gender/%			NS
Male	31.6	20.0	
Female	68.4	80.0	
Performance time/min	19.63 ±3.87	17.35 ±3.13	0.05

NS: No significant.

Table 17 shows the differences in the HRV parameters between the two groups at baseline (PRE), at the 20 – 25 min from the starting of smelling period and after the inhalation period (POST).

Table 17 HRV parameters (M ± SD) in the three HRV session recordings for the two groups

HRV parameters	CON (*N* = 17)	EXP (*N* = 20)	Total (*N* = 37)	*p* value
RRmean/ms				
PRE	854.64 ±118.91	870.10 ±92.10	863.00 ±104.03	<0.001[a]
20 – 25min	865.35 ±114.52	884.85 ±107.01	875.89 ±109.40	
POST	896.88 ±112.69	907.35 ±103.02	902.54 ±106.17	
HR/bpm				
PRE	71.50 ±9.73	69.70 ±7.65	70.58 ±8.59	<0.001[b]
20 – 25min	69.41 ±7.99	67.83 ±7.65	68.60 ±7.76	
POST	67.77 ±8.09	66.89 ±7.27	67.32 ±7.59	

续 表

HRV parameters	CON(N=17)	EXP(N=20)	Total(N=37)	*p* value
SDRR/ms				
PRE	45. 64 ±14. 19	54. 10 ±21. 76	50. 21 ±18. 91	0. 05 *
20 –25min	50. 47 ±16. 88	48. 45 ±16. 84	49. 37 ±16. 65	
POST	57. 76 ±22. 40	56. 90 ±23. 96	57. 29 ±22. 94	
RMSSD/ms				
PRE	26. 58 ±8. 50	33. 30 ±17. 90	30. 21 ±14. 59	0. 02 *
20 –25min	31. 23 ±8. 37	32. 65 ±21. 07	32. 00 ±16. 31	
POST	32. 94 ±11. 96	32. 20 ±13. 67	32. 54 ±12. 74	
LF/HF				
PRE	4. 17 ±4. 21	4. 36 ±5. 48	4. 27 ±4. 87	NS
20 –25min	5. 53 ±6. 04	3. 04 ±2. 49	4. 18 ±4. 59	
POST	5. 73 ±7. 12	3. 45 ±1. 88	4. 50 ±5. 07	
LF/ms^2				
PRE	1013. 05 ±1036. 89	1222. 05 ±1426. 21	1126. 02 ±1250. 01	0. 05 *
20 –25min	990. 94 ±731. 01	739. 15 ±605. 55	854. 83 ±668. 74	
POST	1514. 35 ±1695. 93	1025. 20 ±737. 48	1249. 94 ±275. 31	
HF/ms^2				
PRE	258. 52 ±156. 12	498. 30 ±560. 25	388. 13 ±437. 22	0. 02 *
20 –25min	266. 58 ±165. 24	576. 45 ±1066. 77	434. 08 ±798. 28	
POST	346，29 ±218. 50	393. 15 ±367. 22	371. 62 ±304. 88	
VLF/ms^2				
PRE	779. 00 ±652. 38	1258. 25 ±1052. 01	1038. 05 ±12. 08	0. 058[c]
20 –25min	1167. 76 ±986. 78	932. 75 ±663. 68	1040. 73 ±824. 22	
POST	1815. 76 ±1949. 89	1957. 55 ±2182. 60	1892. 40 ±2051. 62	

续 表

HRV parameters	CON($N=17$)	EXP($N=20$)	Total($N=37$)	p value
LFnu/%				
PRE	71. 11 ± 15. 42	69. 50 ± 17. 92	70. 24 ± 16. 61	0. 08[c]
20 – 25min	74. 64 ± 14. 81	66. 20 ± 18. 26	70. 08 ± 17. 08	
POST	70. 94 ± 20. 81	73. 10 ± 11. 88	72. 10 ± 16. 37	
HFnu/%				
PRE	28. 22 ± 15. 42	30. 50 ± 17. 92	29. 75 ± 16. 61	0. 08[c]
20 – 25min	25. 35 ± 14. 81	33. 80 ± 18. 26	29. 91 ± 17. 08	
POST	29. 05 ± 20. 81	26. 90 ± 11. 85	27. 89 ± 16. 37	

* Significant differences between the two groups. [a]Total differences for all sample: POST > PRE. [b]Total differences for all sample: PRE > POST. [c] Trend to significant differences between the two groups. NS: no significance.

An analysis of variance according to a general linear model (GLM) shows differences between the two groups in terms of evolution throughout the three stages of the session (PRE, 20 – 25 min, and POST) for the following HRV spectral parameters: LF, such that EXP shows a larger LF decrease between PRE and 20 – 25 min than CON, and CON shows a larger LF increase between 20 – 25 min and POST than EXP[$p = 0.05$; see Figure 33 (A)]. HF, such that EXP shows a larger HF decrease between 20 – 25 min and POST than CON, meanwhile CON shows an HF increase in this stage[$p = 0.02$; see Figure 33 (B)]. Figure 33[part (C) and (D)] shows the differences between groups with trend to significance for HFnu($p = 0.08$) and LFnu($p = 0.08$). VLF parameter also shows a trend towards statistical significance($p = 0.058$). GLM analysis shows differences between the two groups for the time domain HRV parameters: SDRR[$p = 0.05$; Figure 33 (E)] and RMSSD[$p = 0.019$; Figure 33 (F)]. There were no significant differences between the two groups for LF/HF, RRmean and heart rate(HR) mean.

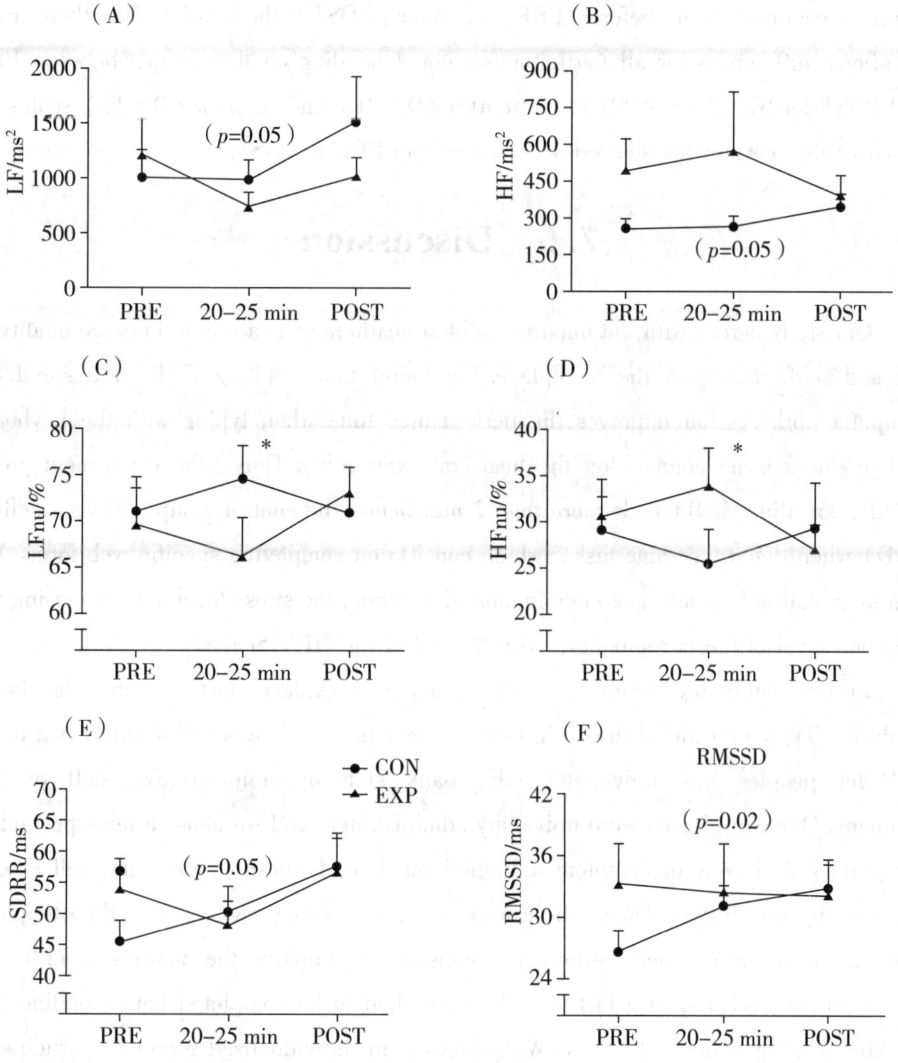

Figure 33 Comparison of HRV parameters during the smelling period [between the two groups at baseline (PRE), at the 20 – 25min period and after the inhalation period (POST)]

(A) low frequency band (LF); (B) high frequency band (HF); (C) LF values expressed in normalized units (LFnu; $*p = 0.08$); (D) HF values expressed in normalized units (HFnu; $*p = 0.08$); (E) standard deviation of all RR intervals (SDRR); (F) root mean square of differences of successive RR intervals (RMSSD).

There were no differences in the questionnaires scorings between the two groups in terms of evolution from before (PRE) to after (POST) the session. But there were significant differences for all participants, not depending on the group, between PRE and POST for STAI($p<0.001$), *tension*($p<0.001$) and *vigor*($p<0.015$) scales. In all cases the participants showed a decrease from PRE to POST.

7.6 Discussion

Our study agrees with the importance of aromatherapy as a way to improve quality of life and performance in the workplace. We found that smelling CAB in a simulated computer work session improves the performance time when typing with the keyboard and produces some changes on the heart rate variability. Thus, the experiment group (EXP, smelling CAB) ends more than 2 min before the control group (CON, smelling PAD) when doing the same task, which consists on completing specific web forms. We aim to explain this result as a combination of reducing the stress level and increasing the attention level of the participants, with the aid of the HRV analysis.

In our study we chose a very common workplace task in the developed countries. Typing on the keyboard in front of a computer during a full workday is a usual task for peoples like university staff, bank staff or administrative staff of any company. Our participants were university administrators and we chose a non-specialized computer task. It was to complete a limited number of questionnaires and self-reports about their own lifestyle. Thus, there were no right or wrong answers and all participants knew the answers. The best performance consisted of thinking the answers quickly and typing on the keyboard in a fast way. All items had to be completed before ending and clicking the last option ("Save"). We promised an individualized report to participants about their lifestyle and all of them completed the items with coherent answers. We randomly distributed the participants to two groups, so they were balanced in terms of mental and typing agility. In these conditions, we have to attribute the performance improvement of EXP (more than 2 min better than CON) showed in our results to the aromatherapy effects (smelling CAB).

The job stress-related problems are currently increasing and potentially affecting employee performance and personal health (Embriaco, Papazian, Kentishe-Barnes, *et* al., 2007). We can find studies about relieving mental load in work places through strategies such as analyzing the exercise effects on autonomic balance (Moreno, Ramos-Castro, Movellan, *et al.*, 2015) or about the effects of aromatherapy in alleviating work-related stress (Liu, Cheng, Wang, *et al.*, 2015). A growing number of studies described the efficacy of aromatherapy treatment in this field (Liu, Lin, Chang, 2013). However, few studies examined the effects of aromatherapy directly on work performance through the autonomic balance. In our study, we have contributed to this using HRV analysis to explain the performance improvement in experiment group by a stress reduction due to the aromatherapy effect.

This stress reduction could be explained by a specific effect on the autonomic nervous system. For this purpose, in our study we analyzed in three 5 min periods: before smelling, 20 min after inhalation began, and after the inhalation period. The main findings reveal significant differences between both groups in HF-related and LF-related parameters. These indexes have been used to reflect primarily sympathetic and parasympathetic influences (Matsumoto, Asakura, Hayashi, 2013). The larger LF decrease between PRE and 20 – 25 min in EXP could be explained by a specific effect of smelling CAB reducing the sympathetic activity during the task performance. Otherwise, the sympathetic effect could be effective during the last session period, where CON showed a larger LF increase than that of EXP. In this last period (between 20 – 25 min and POST) the parasympathetic activity (showed by HF) is different in both groups. We can see this same trend for the standardized parameters. Thus, the most important aromatherapy effect is the increased parasympathetic activity (HF and HFnu increases) for EXP between PRE and 20 – 25 period, combined with a decline of the sympathetic activity (LF and LFnu decreases) for this group in the same period. These changes could produce a sympathetic/parasympathetic balance of the ANS improving the attention control and facilitating the performance. In addition, the significant decrease of SDRR parameter in EXP during the task (PRE and 20 – 25 min) means a minor cardiac variability than CON, and could be interpreted as an increase of arousal. This higher arousal could permit EXP to pay more attention to the task and improve the performance. Thus, smelling CAB could improve the mental and emotional condition in terms of attentiveness and alertness.

We also analyzed the cognitive levels of anxiety and mood state as stress symptoms in our study. But we did not find differences between two groups. We found significant differences for all participants for anxiety scores (STAI) and psychological tension (POMS). They showed less anxiety values after the session, but these global results were expected because they had just performed a theoretical stressful task. Maybe we would need more than one aromatherapy session to obtain more cognitive anxiety reduction in EXP. But, what is the mechanism of action underlying the performance improvement effect of smelling CAB? Aromatherapy could drive autonomic nervous activity towards a balanced state (Chang, Shen, 2011). This balance could be explained by the combined action of CAB main components. On the one hand, some of these components have sedative effects, such as linalyl acetate and linalool, which could induce changes on the parasympathetic activity (Igarashi, 2013). In this sense, Kuroda, Inoue, Ito, *et al.* (2005) found that HF power increased more significantly at 21 min after a 6 min olfactory stimulation of linalool. In the same line, we found changes at 20 – 25 min after starting the smelling period. Thus, CAB seems to have an increasing effect on parasympathetic activity in EXP (HF and HFnu) from 0 min to 20 – 25 min and a clearly higher decreasing effect on parasympathetic activity in EXP (HF and HFnu) from 20 – 25 min to POST. Meanwhile, CON decreased HF and HFnu values in POST period. On the other hand, myrcene is another component in CAB that could have some activation effects by stimulating the sympathetic activity (Herz, 2009). Myrcene, a kind of monoterpene (1.3% – 2.12%), could possibly be related to the release of norepinephrine, a neurotransmitter linked with the sympathetic activity stimulation (Chang, Shen, 2011). This could help to explain our results as an increase of the arousal levels in EXP. Similar results were found with pepper oil smelling, which induce an increase in adrenaline concentration, while inhalation of rose oil decreased the adrenaline level. The same stimulating effects of essential oils on sympathetic and parasympathetic activity have been reported, e. g. estragon oil or grapefruit oil. These essential oils, as pepper oil, consist of some components, such as limonene, pinene or methyl chavicol, which possibly mediate the stimulating effect on sympathetic activity. Furthermore, alcohols such as citronellol, geraniol, nerol and patchouli alcohol were detected in rose oil and patchouli oil, which induce inhibition of parasympathetic activity(Haze, Sakai, Gozu, 2002).

The olfactory system interactions could be another mechanism of action to explain the effects of CAB through an interaction with central nervous system structures (e. g. hypothalamic, limbic, thalamic), which control the level of autonomic and behavioral arousal(Bowers, 2006). The olfactory neuroanatomy is intertwined, via extensive reciprocal axonal connections, with primary emotion areas including the amygdala, hippocampus, and orbitofrontal cortex and other parts of the limbic system. The odor molecules of essential oils are transmitted to the brain by olfactory sensory neurons in the nasal cavity; thus, they stimulate smell-memory work and influence memory, thoughts, and emotions (Stea, Berardi, de Pasquale, 2014). Further studies are needed to evaluate the olfactory system interactions and another possible action mechanism underlying the workplace stress and performance improvement effect of aromatherapy.

7.7 Conclusion

Our study confirms that aromatherapy (inhaling *Petitgrain* essential oil) can improve the performance in the workplace. The most important aromatherapy effect is the increased parasympathetic activity for EXP between PRE and 20 – 25 period, combined with a decline of the sympathetic activity for this group in the same period. These changes could produce a sympathetic/parasympathetic balance of the ANS improving the attention control and facilitating the performance. This balance could be explained by a combined action of the *Petitgrain* main components (like linalyl acetate, linalool or myrcene). On the one hand, some of these components have sedative effects, which could induce changes on the parasympathetic activity. On the other hand, other components could have some activation effects by stimulating the sympathetic activity. The final effect could be an improvement of the mental and emotional condition by a combination of reducing the stress level and increasing the arousal level of the participants in terms of attentiveness and alertness.

8 Conclusion

1. This book confirms that aromatherapy (inhaling essential oils) can improve performance in the workplace, and help to manage negative emotions and increase attention level in academic and workplace situations.

2. Our results confirm that inhalation of essential oils produces this effect by balancing the sympathetic/parasympathetic system of the autonomic nervous system. HRV analysis is a good marker of this effect.

3. Inhalation of *Petitgrain* essential oil reduces stress and improves performance in the workplace(Study 2). AR improves the performance time when typing with the keyboard in a simulated computer work session and produces some changes improving HRV.

4. Inhalation of *Sweet basil* essential oil reduces academic anxiety and improves study concentration of university students(Study 1). AR in a short session or with an aromatic necklace every day during one month produces emotional and HRV changes on participants.

5. Inhalation of essential oils has its most acute effects at 20 – 25 min after starting inhaling, both with *Petitgrain* and *Sweet basil* oils. It means it will be enough to program 30 min sessions with a short-time effect to reduce negative emotions and improve performance in academic and workplace situations.

6. AR has short-term efficacy(one-hour) to reduce negative emotions and improve performance in academic and workplace situations, and long-term efficacy(one-month) to reduce negative emotions in academic situations.

7. This ANS balance can be explained by a combined action of the *Petitgrain* and *Sweet basil* main components. Some of them have sedative effects, which can induce changes on the parasympathetic activity, and others have activation effects, which stimulate the sympathetic activity. The final effect can be an improvement of the mental and emotional condition by a combination of reducing stress level and increasing arousal level of the participants in terms of attentiveness and alertness.

8. We can also explain our results according to TCM. Essential oils can work through a truly holistic therapy, taking into account the mind, the body and the spirit of the person. Essential oils can connect with our body and help it to find the best way to solve its needs. The relaxing effects(parasympathetic activity) can be related to Yin and the activation effects(sympathetic activity) can be related to Yang.

References

Baik J S, Kim S S, Lee J A, et al., 2008. Chemical composition and biological activities of essential oils extracted from Korean endemic citrus species. *Journal of Microbiology and Biotechnology*, 18(1): 74–79.

Bakkali F, Averbeck S, Averbeck D, et al., 2008. Biological effects of essential oils: A review. *Food and Chemical Toxicology*, 46: 446–475.

Blanck T J, Dugan K, Kline R, et al., 2016. Lavender fleur oil and unscented oil can reduce preoperative anxiety in breast surgery patients. *Journal of Clinical Anesthesia*. doi: 10.1016.

Boeree C G. *Viktor Frankl: 1905–1997*, Shippensburg University.

Bowers L J, 2006. To what extent does aromatherapy use in palliative cancer care improve quality of life and reduce levels of psychological distress? A literatura review. *International Journal of Aromatherapy*, 16(1): 27–35.

Cervantes J C, Rodas G, Capdevila L, 2009. Heart-rate variability and precompetitive anxiety in swimmers. *Psicothema*, 21(4): 531–536.

Chamine I, Oken B S, 2016. Aroma effects on physiologic and cognitive function following acute stress: A mechanism investigation. *Journal of Alternative and Complementary Medicine*, 22(9): 712–721.

Chang K M, Shen C W, 2011. Aromatherapy benefits autonomic nervous system regulation for elementary school faculty in Taiwan. *Evidence-based Complementary and Alternative Medicine*, 946537. doi: 10.1155/2011/946537.

Chien L W, Cheng S L, Liu C F, 2012. The effect of lavender aromatherapy on autonomic nervous system in midlife women with insomnia. *Evidence-based Complementary and Alternative Medicine*. doi: 10.1155/2012/740813.

Conder R L, Conder A A, 2014. Heart rate variability interventions for concussion and rehabilitation. *Front Psychol*, 5: 890. doi: 10. 3389/fpsyg. 2014. 00890.

Cooke B, Ernst E, 2000. Aromatherapy: A systematic review. *The British Journal of General Practice*, 50(455): 493 -496.

Davis P, 2005. *Aromatherapy an a - z: the most comprehensive guide to aromatherapy ever published*, Random House.

Deng L Y, 2001. *Chinese Acupuncturee-Moxibustion.* World Health Organization Regional Office for South-East Asia New Delhi. 9290222247.

Dong H G, Zhang X R, 2001. *An Overview of Traditional Chinese Medicine.* World Health Organization Regional Office for South-East Asia New Delhi. 9290222247.

Eguchi E, Funakubo N, Tomooka K, et al. , 2016. The effects of aroma foot massage on blood pressure and anxiety in Japanese community-dwelling men and women: A crossover randomized controlled trial. *PLoS One*, 11(3).

Embriaco N, Papazian L, Kentishe-Barnes N, et al. , 2007. Burnout syndrome among critical care healthcare workers. *Current Opinion in Critical Care*, 13 (5): 482 -488.

Franchomme P, Jollois R, Penoel D, 2001. *L'Aromatherapie Exactement.* Paris, France: Roger Jollois: 486.

Haze S, Sakai K, Gozu Y, 2002. Effect of fragrance inhalation on sympathetic activity in normal adults. *The Japanese Journal of Pharmacology*, 90(3): 247 -253.

Herz R S, 2009. Aromatherapy facts and fictions: A scientific analysis of olfactory effects on mood, physiology and behavior. *The International Journal of Neuroscience*, 119(2): 263 -290.

Hosseini S-A, Heydari A, Vakili M, et al, 2016. Effect of lavender essence inhalation on the level of anxiety and blood cortisol in candidates for open - heart surgery. *Iran J Nurs Midwifery Res*, 21(4): 397 -401.

Hu J Q, Liu B Y, 2012. The basic theory, diagnostic, and therapeutic system of traditional Chinese medicine and the challenges they bring to statistics. *Statistics in Medicine*, 31(7): 602 -605.

Huang L, Capdevila L, 2017. Aromatherapy improves work performance through balancing the autonomic nervous system. *J Altern Complement Med*, 23 (3): 214 -

221. doi: 10.1089.

Igarashi M, Ikei H, Song C, et al., 2014. Effects of olfactory stimulation with rose and orange oil on prefrontal cortex activity. *Complementary Therapies in Medicine*, 22(6): 1027 – 1031.

Igarashi T, 2013. Physical and psychologic effects of aromatherapy inhalation on pregnant women: A randomized controlled trial. *The Journal of Alternative and Complementary Medicine*, 19: 805 – 810.

Janes S E, Price C S, Thomas D, 2005. Essential oil poisoning: Nacetylcysteine for eugenol-induced hepatic failure and analysis of a national database. *European Journal of Pediatrics*, 164(8): 520 – 522.

Jänig W, 1989. The autonomic nervous system. *Human Physiology*: 333 – 370.

Joshi R K, 2014. Chemical composition and antimicrobial activity of the essential oil of Ocimum basilicum L. (sweet basil) from Western Ghats of North West Karnataka, India. *Anc Sci Life*, 4(3): 200 – 214.

Kamatou G P P, Makunga N P, Ramogola W P N, et al, 2008. South African Salvia species: a review of biological activities and phytochemistry. *J Ethnopharmacol.* doi: 10.1016/j.jep.2008.06.030.

Koulivand P H, Khaleghi Ghadiri M, Gorji A, 2013. Lavender and the nervous system. *Evidence-based Complementary and Alternative Medicine*: *eCAM*, 2013: 681304.

Krusemark E A, Novak L R, Gitelman D R, et al., 2013. When the sense of smell meets emotion: Anxiety-state-dependent olfactory processing and neural circuitry adaptation. *The Journal of Neuroscience*, 33(39): 15324 – 15332.

Kudo N, Shinohara H, Kodama H, 2014. Heart rate variability biofeedback intervention for reduction of psychological stress during the early postpartum period. *Applied Psychophysiology and Biofeedback*, 39(3 – 4): 203 – 211.

Kuroda K, Inoue N, Ito Y, et al., 2005. Sedative effects of the jasmine tea odor and(R)-(-)-linalool, one of its major odor components, on autonomic nerve activity and mood states. *European Journal of Applied Physiology*, 95(2 – 3): 107 – 114.

Lehrner J, Christine Eckersberger, Walla P, et al, 2000. Ambient odor of orange in a dental office reduces anxiety and improves mood in female patients. *Physiology & Behavior*, 71(1 – 2): 83 – 86.

Li Z J, Xu C B, 2011. The fundamental theory of traditional Chinese medicine and the consideration in its research strategy. *Frontiers of Medicine*, 5(2): 208 - 211.

Liu S H, Cheng D C, Wang J J, et al., 2015. Effects of moderate exercise on relieving mental load of elementary school teachers. *Evidence-based Complementary and Alternative Medicine*, 192680. doi: 10.1155/2015/192680.

Liu S H, Lin T H, Chang K M, 2013. The physical effects of aromatherapy in alleviating work-related stress on elementary school teachers in Taiwan. *Evidence-based Complementary and Alternative Medicine.* doi: 10.1155/2013/853809.

Luque-Casado A, Zabala M, Morales E, et al., 2013. Cognitive performance and heart rate variability: The influence of fitness level. *PLoS One.* https://doi.org/10.1371/journal.pone.0056935.

Lu A P, Jia H W, Cheng X, et al., 2004. Theory of traditional Chinese medicine and therapeutic method of diseases. *World Journal of Gastroenterology*, 10 (13): 1854 - 1856.

Małachowska B, Fendler W, Pomykała A, et al., 2016. Essential oils reduce autonomous response to pain sensation during self-monitoring of blood glucose among children with diabetes. *Journal of Pediatric Endocrinology and Metabolism.* doi: 10.1515/jpem - 2014 - 0361.

Marchese A, Orhan I E, Daglia M, et al., 2016. Antibacterial and antifungal activities of thymol: A brief review of the literature. *Food Chemistry*, 201: 402 - 414.

Matsumoto T, Asakura H, Hayashi T, 2013. Does lavender aromatherapy alleviate premenstrual emotional symptoms?: A randomized crossover trial. *BioPsychoSocial Medicine*, 7: 12.

McCorry L K, 2007. Physiology of the autonomic nervous system. *American Journal of Pharmaceutical Education*, 71(4): 78.

Moreno J, Ramos-Castro J, Movellan J, et al., 2015. Facial video-based photoplethysmography to detect HRV at rest. *International Journal of Sports Medicine*, 36(6): 474 - 480.

Moreno J, Ramos-Castro J, Rodas G, et al., 2015. Individual profiles of recovery in basketball players. *The Spanish Journal of Psychology*, 18. doi: 10.1017/sjp.2015.23.

Parrado E, Garcia M A, Ramos J, et al, 2010. Comparison of omega wave system and polar S810i to detect R－R intervals at rest. *International Journal of Sports Medicine*, 110 (2): 699－713.

Patrcia D, 1992. *Aromatherapy An A-Z: The Most Comprehensive Guide to Aromatherapy Ever Published.* Penguin Random House, UK.

Peana A T, D'Aquila P S, Panin F, et al., 2002. Anti-inflammatory activity of linalool and linalyl acetate constituents of essential oils. *Phytomedicine*, 9 (8): 721－726.

Peana A T, Marzocco S, Popolo A, et al., 2006. (-)-Linalool inhibits in vitro NO formation: Probable involvement in the antinociceptive activity of this monoterpene compound. *Life Sciences*, 78(7): 719－723.

Pierre-Marie L, Gilles G, Jean-Didier V, 2005. Information processing in the mammalian olfactory system. *Physiological Reviews*, 85(1): 281－317.

Price S, Price L, 1995. *Aromatherapy for Health Professionals.* New York: Churchill Livingstone.

Pryia R M, Blessed B P, Nija S, 2014. Chemical composition, antibacterial and antioxidant profile of essential oil from Murraya koenigii(L.) leaves. *Avicenna Journal of Phytomedicine*, 4: 200－214.

Reddy M S, 2010. Depression: The Disorder and the Burden. *Indian Journal of Psychological Medicine*, 32(1): 1－2.

Reyes del Paso G A, Langewitz W, Mulder L J M, et al, 2013. The utility of low frequency heart rate variability as an index of sympathetic cardiac tone: A review with emphasis on a reanalysis of previous studies. *Psychophysiology*, 50: 477－487.

Robin O, Alaoui-Ismaïli O, Dittmar A, et al., 1999. Basic emotions evoked by eugenol odor differ according to the dental experience: A neurovegetative analysis. *Chemical Senses*, 24(3): 327－335.

Robins J L, 1999. The science and art of aromatherapy. *Journal of Holistic Nursing*, 17(1): 5－17.

Ruan W J, Lai M D, Zhou J G, 2006. Anticancer effects of Chinese herbal medicine, science or myth? *Journal of Zhejiang University SCIENCE B*, 7(12): 1006－1014.

Saeki Y, 2000. The effect of foot-bath with or without the essential oil of lavender on the autonomic nervous system: A randomized trial. *International Journal of Aromatherapy*, 10(1 –2): 57 –61.

Satou T, Chikama M, Chikama Y, et al. , 2013. Effect of aromatherapy massage on elderly patients under long-term hospitalization in Japan. *Journal of alternative and complementary medicine(New York, N. Y.)*, 19(3): 235 –237.

Schmidt R F, Thews G, 1989. *Human Physiology* (2 ed). Berlin: Springer Verlag: 333 –370.

Schnaubelt K, 1998. *Advanced Aromatherapy: The Science of Essential Oil Therapy*. Healing Arts Press, UK.

Sfeir J, Lefrançois C, Baudoux D, et al. , 2013. In vitro antibacterial activity of essential oils against Streptococcus pyogenes. *Evidence-Based Complementary and Alternative Medicine*. http: //dx. doi. org/10. 1155/2013/269161.

Shacham S, 1983. A shortened version of the Profile of Mood States. *Journal of Personality Assessment*, 47(3): 305 –306.

Sharma D, Paudel B H, Khadka R, et al. , 2015. Time domain and frequency domain analysis of heart rate variability in elite Nepalese football players. *International Journal of Biomedical Research*, 6(9). doi: 10. 7439/ijbr. v6i9. 2413.

Shin E S, Seo K H, Lee S H, et al. , 2016. Massage with or without aromatherapy for symptom relief in people with cancer. *Cochrane Database of Systematic Reviews*. doi: 10. 1002/14651858. CD009873. pub3.

Shin L M, Liberzon I, 2010. The neurocircuitry of fear, stress, and anxiety disorders. *Neuropsychopharmacology*, 35(1): 169 –191.

Shu Q, Wang H, Litscher D, et al. , 2016. Acupuncture and moxibustion have different effects on fatigue by regulating the autonomic nervous system: A pilot controlled clinical trial. *Akupunktur & Aurikulomedizin*, 42(4): 11.

Solgi M, Ghorbanpour M, 2014. Application of essential oils and their biological effects on extending the shelf-life and quality of horticultural crops. *Trakia Journal of Sciences*, 12(2): 198 –210.

Souto-Maior F N, de Carvalho F L, de Morais L C, et al. , 2011. Anxiolytic-like effects of inhaled linalool oxide in experimental mouse anxiety models. *Pharmacology*, *biochemistry*, *and behavior*, 100(2): 259 – 263.

Spielberger C D, 2010. State-trait anxiety inventory (" Self-Evaluation Questionnaire").

Stea S, Beraudi A, de Pasquale D, 2014. Essential oils for complementary treatment of surgical patients: State of the art. *Evidence-based Complementary and Alternative Medicine.* doi: 10.1155/2014/726341.

Taelman J, Vandeput S, Vlemincx E, et al., 2011. Instantaneous changes in heart rate regulation due to mental load in simulated office work. *European Journal of Applied Physiology*, 111(7): 1497 – 1505.

Task Force of the European Society of Cardiology and the North American Society of Pacing and Electrophysiology, 1996. Heart rate variability: Standards of measurement, physiological interpretation and clinical use. *European Heart Journal*, 17: 354 – 381.

Tortoriello J, Romero O, 1992. Plants used by Mexican traditional medicine with presumable sedative properties: An ethnobotanical approach. *Archives of Medical Research*, 23(3): 111 – 116.

Vázquez F M, Suarez M A, Pérez A, 1997. Medicinal plants used in the Barros Area, Badajoz Province, Spain. *Journal of Ethnopharmacology*, 55(2): 81 – 85.

Zhou C C, 2008. *The Illustrated Book of Traditional Chinese Cultivation of Health.* New World Press.

Alternative-medicine, 2016. https://healdove.com/alternativeemedicine.

How the olfactory system works, 2011. http://www.gridgit.com/postpic/2010/11/howetheeolfactoryesystemeworks_502244.jpg.

Southern California Acupuncture, 2016. http://www.southerncaliforniaacupuncture.com.

http://www.taozhy.com/ShuJuKu/XueWei/104.thtml.

http://alternativeresourcesdirectory.com/news/what-are-the-meridians.

Appendixes: Original Questionnaires Used in the Study

Laboratori de Psicologia de l'Esport, UAB

Aromatherapy Study

Researcher: Huang Lin

Data: ____/____/____ **Hora:________**

DNI: ________________ (Si no recordes el DNI, identifica't amb el **NIU:** __________________)

Sexe: O Dona O Home **Data de Naixement: ____/____/19__**

Edat: __________ **Pes:** _____**kg.** **Alçada:** ______**cm.**

Instruccions

Si us plau, llegeix acuradament les diferents instruccions de cada qüestionari i contesta sincerament totes les preguntes, sense deixar-ne cap en blanc.

Control de la HRV

INSTRUCCIONES:

A continuación, te haremos algunas preguntas sobre aspectos que pueden influir en los resultados del estudio.

1. ¿Has tomado alguna medicación durante las últimas 24 horas?	☐ Sí ☐ No ¿Cuál/es? ____________ ____________ ____________ ¿A qué hora? ____________
2. ¿Has hecho actividad física durante las últimas 20 horas?	☐ Sí ☐ No ¿Qué tipo? ____________ ¿A qué hora? ____________ ¿Durante cuánto tiempo? ____________ ¿Cuántas horas han pasado desde que acabaste la actividad? ____________
3. ¿Has tomado cafeína hoy?	☐ Sí ☐ No ¿Cuántas horas hace? ____________
4. ¿Has fumado hoy?	☐ Sí ☐ No ¿Cuántas horas hace del último cigarro? ____________
5. ¿Has tomado alguna bebida alcohólica durante las últimas 10 horas?	☐ Sí ☐ No
6. ¿Has realizado alguna comida copiosa en las últimas tres horas?	☐ Sí ☐ No
7. ¿Has comido alguna cosa en la última hora?	☐ Sí ☐ No
8. ¿Cuántas horas has dormido esta noche? ____________ ________ ¿Crees que el tu sueño ha sido de calidad?	☐ Sí ☐ No

Su Salud y Bienestar

Las preguntas que siguen se refieren a lo que usted piensa sobre su salud. Sus respuestas permitirán saber cómo se encuentra usted y hasta qué punto es capaz de hacer sus actividades habituales.
Gracias por contestar a estas preguntas.

Para cada una de las siguientes preguntas, por favor marque con una ☒ la casilla que mejor corresponda a su respuesta.

1. En general, usted diría que su salud es:

Excelente	Muy buena	Buena	Regular	Mala
☐ 1	☐ 2	☐ 3	☐ 4	☐ 5

2. Las siguientes preguntas se refieren a actividades o cosas que usted podría hacer en un día normal. Su salud actual, ¿le limita para hacer esas actividades o cosas? Si es así, ¿cuánto?

	Sí, me limita mucho	Sí, me limita un poco	No, no me limita nada
a Esfuerzos moderados, como mover una mesa, pasar la aspiradora, jugar a los bolos o caminar más de 1 hora.	☐ 1	☐ 2	☐ 3
b Subir varios pisos por la escalera.	☐ 1	☐ 2	☐ 3

3. Durante <u>las 4 últimas semanas</u>, ¿con qué frecuencia ha tenido alguno de los siguientes problemas en su trabajo o en sus actividades cotidianas, <u>a causa de su salud física</u>?

	Siempre	Casi siempre	Algunas veces	Sólo alguna vez	Nunca
a ¿Hizo menos de lo que hubiera querido hacer?	☐ 1	☐ 2	☐ 3	☐ 4	☐ 5
b ¿Tuvo que dejar de hacer algunas tareas en su trabajo o en sus actividades cotidianas?	☐ 1	☐ 2	☐ 3	☐ 4	☐ 5

4. Durante <u>las 4 últimas semanas</u>, ¿con qué frecuencia ha tenido alguno de los siguientes problemas en su trabajo o en sus actividades cotidianas, a causa de <u>algún problema emocional</u> (como estar triste, deprimido, o nervioso)?

	Siempre	Casi siempre	Algunas veces	Sólo alguna vez	Nunca
a ¿Hizo menos de lo que hubiera querido hacer por algún problema emocional?	☐ 1	☐ 2	☐ 3	☐ 4	☐ 5
b ¿Hizo su trabajo o sus actividades cotidianas menos cuidadosamente que de costumbre, por algún problema emocional?	☐ 1	☐ 2	☐ 3	☐ 4	☐ 5

5. Durante las <u>4 últimas semanas</u>, ¿hasta qué punto <u>el dolor</u> le ha dificultado su trabajo habitual (incluido el trabajo fuera de casa y las tareas domésticas)?

Nada	Un poco	Regular	Bastante	Mucho
☐ 1	☐ 2	☐ 3	☐ 4	☐ 5

6. Las preguntas que siguen se refieren a cómo se ha sentido y cómo le han ido las cosas durante las 4 últimas semanas. En cada pregunta responda lo que se parezca más a cómo se ha sentido usted. Durante las últimas 4 semanas ¿con qué frecuencia...

	Siempre	Casi siempre	Algunas veces	Sólo alguna vez	Nunca
Se sintió calmado y tranquilo?	□ 1	□ 2	□ 3	□ 4	□ 5
Tuvo mucha energía?	□ 1	□ 2	□ 3	□ 4	□ 5
Se sintió desanimado y deprimido?	□ 1	□ 2	□ 3	□ 4	□ 5

7. Durante las 4 últimas semanas, ¿con qué frecuencia la salud física o los problemas emocionales le han dificultado sus actividades sociales (como visitar a los amigos o familiares)?

Siempre	Casi siempre	Algunas veces	Sólo alguna vez	Nunca
□ 1	□ 2	□ 3	□ 4	□ 5

STAI A-E

(PRE and POS)

INSTRUCCIONES

A continuación encontrará unas frases que se utilizan corrientemente para describirse uno a sí mismo.

Lea cada frase y señale la puntuación de 0 a 3 que indique mejor **CÓMO SE SIENTE USTED AHORA MISMO, en este momento.** No hay respuestas buenas ni malas. No emplee demasiado tiempo en cada frase y conteste señalando la respuesta que mejor describa su situación presente.

0	NADA
1	ALGO
2	BASTANTE
3	MUCHO

	Nada	Algo	Bastante	Mucho
1. Me siento calmado.	0	1	2	3
2. Me siento seguro.	0	1	2	3
3. Estoy tenso.	0	1	2	3
4. Estoy contrariado.	0	1	2	3
5. Me siento cómodo (estoy a gusto).	0	1	2	3
6. Me siento alterado.	0	1	2	3
7. Estoy preocupado por posibles desgracias futuras.	0	1	2	3
8. Me siento descansado.	0	1	2	3
9. Me siento angustiado.	0	1	2	3
10. Me siento confortable.	0	1	2	3
11. Tengo confianza en mí mismo.	0	1	2	3
12. Me siento nervioso.	0	1	2	3
13. Estoy desasosegado.	0	1	2	3
14. Me siento muy "atado" (como oprimido).	0	1	2	3
15. Estoy relajado.	0	1	2	3
16. Me siento satisfecho.	0	1	2	3
17. Estoy preocupado.	0	1	2	3
18. Me siento aturdido y sobreexcitado.	0	1	2	3
19. Me siento alegre.	0	1	2	3
20. En este momento me siento bien.	0	1	2	3

Estado de Ánimo.	*(PRE and POS)*
INSTRUCCIONES: A continuación aparece una lista de palabras utilizadas por la gente para describir sus sensaciones. Lee cada palabra o frase y marca el número apropiado que aparece a la derecha para indicar ***cómo te sientes en este momento***.	
En este momento me siento:	**Nada Algo Bastante Mucho**
1. Tenso/a	0 1 2 3 4 5 6 7 8 9 10
2. Enfadado/a	0 1 2 3 4 5 6 7 8 9 10
3. Agotado/a	0 1 2 3 4 5 6 7 8 9 10
4. Infeliz	0 1 2 3 4 5 6 7 8 9 10
5. Activo/a	0 1 2 3 4 5 6 7 8 9 10
6. Enérgico/a	0 1 2 3 4 5 6 7 8 9 10
7. Fatigado/a	0 1 2 3 4 5 6 7 8 9 10
8. Desanimado/a	0 1 2 3 4 5 6 7 8 9 10
9. Nervioso/a	0 1 2 3 4 5 6 7 8 9 10
10. Ansioso/a	0 1 2 3 4 5 6 7 8 9 10
11. Deprimido/a	0 1 2 3 4 5 6 7 8 9 10
12. Furioso/a	0 1 2 3 4 5 6 7 8 9 10
13. De mal genio	0 1 2 3 4 5 6 7 8 9 10
14. Vigoroso/a	0 1 2 3 4 5 6 7 8 9 10
15. Cansado/a	0 1 2 3 4 5 6 7 8 9 10

¿Cómo te sientes hoy? (Escoge "Mal" o "Bien" y un número de la escala)

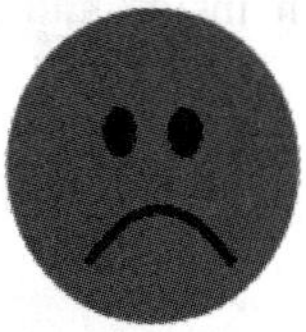

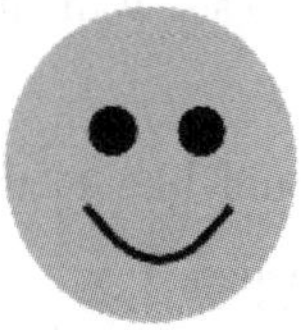

1 2 3 4 5 6 7 8 9 10

Mal **Bien**

Acknowledgment

The research has been a long and hard journey for me. I have put time and efforts on this project and many people have walked the path with me. I appreciate the efforts of all of them:

First, I would like to thank Professor Lluís, who gives me the opportunity to study in Spain and he has trained me to become a researcher at his side for these years. He trusts and teaches me what I need to know as a good psychologist and he also offers me good advice and the helpful support I need to access the doctorate. He did not only train me to become a researcher, but also taught me how to become a good teacher.

I would like to thank Professor Eva as well, who always supported me in my study. She gave me a lot of good advice and helped me improve my study; she has reminded me how to do a basic research and taught me about heathy aspects of cognition of sports. Whenever I need it, she is always willing to help me and she gave me invaluable support to do my pilot study.

I would like to thank my colleagues, especially Jaume, Jordi and Judit with whom I shared both great and difficult moments as professionals and individuals during the course of the thesis. With them I have great memories together both inside and outside the "lab".

I also would like to thank the secretaries of the Service, who always helped me whenever I needed.

I would like to thank my friends Pei, Jia and Mei, who have supported and helped me during difficult times when I had some problems in China.

I would like to thank my family: To my grandmother. You have given me the best care when I was a child, but I did not give you the best care when you left this world;

I believe that my achievement makes you happy. Thank you, grandma, I miss you. To my parents, who supported me unconditionally to ensure that my education helped me to get where I am. To my old sister Yin Huang, who has always been by my side when I needed her. To my dear son Yan Song, thank you for never letting me worry about you, and also helping me with my study. I feel so lucky to be your Mum. Thanks to my cousin Yin Long; without your support I might have not finished my study, I am always happy to talk to you about our life and our dreams. Finally, thanks to my husband, because you take care of all our family, so I can study in Spain without worrying. I love you forever.

I would like to thank Kunming University for helping me to grow and become a real researcher and teacher.

I would like to thank Spain and Spanish people, who are so enthusiastic and friendly; thank you for letting me study here and making me feel less homesick. Spain has become a second homeland to me.

I would like to express my heartfelt gratitude to all those who have helped throughout this long but pleasant journey.

